Paleo Diet Cookbook for Beginners

2 Books in 1| Paleo Gillian's Meal Plan| Complete Guide to Approach The Food Path of Homo Sapiens Safely and Without Stress

By Kaylee Gillian

ISBN: 978-1-80321-510-5 (Paperback)

ISBN: 978-1-80321-511-2 (Hardcover)

Table of Contents

Paleo Diet Cookbook for Men

Paleo Diet Cookbook on a Budget

Paleo Diet Cookbook for Men

Paleo Gillian's Meal Plan| Sculpt Your Body by Following a Carb-Free Eating Plan

By Kaylee Gillian

Chapter 1 -   Introduction

Paleo Diet is based on the idea that even modern men should eat as it was done in the distant past, this not only to ensure a healthy weight but also to keep healthy.

In order to stay healthy, according to Cordain, it is necessary to follow a diet very rich in animal proteins in which carbohydrates are completely excluded except those contained in fruits and vegetables. It is also important to associate to the paleolithic diet a regular physical activity: our ancestors in fact were not sedentary as they had to struggle every day to get the food they needed as they could not buy it easily in markets or supermarkets.

According to the creator, it would be a very simple diet to follow and always suitable, so not only in case you want to lose weight.

Have many small meals and not a few large ones; this also reduces hormonal (insulin) stimulation compared to that caused by larger, more concentrated meals.

Eat red or white meat (even if today's meat is treated compared to millions of years ago and loses many nutritional values compared to the paleolithic one; it is not a coincidence that farm animals are given feed with cereals inside, when they were free, however, they ate what nature had imposed) and carbohydrates taken from fruits and vegetables, avoiding pasta, bread, cookies, rusks, rice and all derivatives of cereals

Dissociate foods correctly, that is avoid mixing different proteins, in this way each food will be better digested and absorbed by the body.

Do physical activity: Paleolithic man went to hunt for food, he did not sit on a sofa watching TV, and made a fight to kill the animal; now instead we go to the supermarket and everything is already ready, so it is very important to do some sport.

With this diet, also associated with a zone diet, I was able to "bring back to the roots" many people in a short time, devastated by dietary regimes that unfortunately today's society imposes on us. Happy re-entry into today's civilization or happy beginning of a new era...paleo!

Chapter 2 -   Breakfast Recipes

1)   Turkey and Cranberry Sandwich

Preparation Time: 5 minutes   **Cooking Time:**   **Servings:1**

Ingredients:

- 2 turkey breast slices, skinless, boneless and roasted
- 2 tablespoons walnuts, toasted and chopped
- 2 slices paleo coconut bread

- 2 tablespoons cranberry chutney
- ¼ cup baby arugula

Directions:

⇒ In a bowl, mix the walnuts with the chutney, stir and spread on one paleo slice of bread.

⇒ Add the turkey slices and the arugula, top with the other slice of bread and serve.

Nutrition: calories 347, fat 12,7, fiber 13,6, carbs 37,4, protein 28,6

2)   Coconut Berry Smoothie

Preparation Time: 5 minutes   **Cooking Time:**   **Servings:2**

Ingredients:

- 2 cups blueberries
- 1 teaspoon lemon zest, grated
- ½ cup coconut milk

- 1 teaspoon cinnamon powder
- 3 cups water

Directions:

⇒ In a blender, combine all the ingredients, pulse well, divide into 2 glasses and serve for breakfast.

Nutrition: calories 222, fat 14,8, fiber 4,9, carbs 24,5, protein 2,5

3)   Lemon Kale Smoothie

Preparation Time: 5 minutes   **Cooking Time:**   **Servings:2**

Ingredients:

- 1 small cucumber, peeled and chopped
- 1 green apple, chopped
- Juice of ½ lemon
- Juice of ½ lime

- 1 tablespoon ginger, finely grated
- 1 cup kale, chopped
- 1 cup coconut water

Directions:

⇒ In a blender, combine all the ingredients, pulse well, divide into 2 glasses and serve for breakfast.

Nutrition: calories 138, fat 1, fiber 5,8, carbs 32,1, protein 3,6

4)   Cabbage and Berry Smoothie

Preparation Time: 5 minutes   **Cooking Time:**   **Servings:2**

Ingredients:

- 1 small red bell pepper, seeded and roughly chopped
- 5 strawberries, halved
- 1 tomato, cut into 4 wedges
- 1 cup red cabbage, chopped

- ½ cup raspberries
- 8 ounces water
- 2 ice cubes for serving

Directions:

⇒ In a blender, combine all the ingredients and pulse well.   ⇒
Divide into glasses and serve.

Nutrition: calories 200, fat 5, fiber 11, carbs 20, protein 9

5) Mint Berry Smoothie

Preparation Time: 10 minutes   Cooking Time: Servings:2

Ingredients:

- 1 and ½ cups kiwi, chopped
- 1 and ½ cups frozen strawberries, chopped
- 8 mint leaves

- 2 cups crushed ice
- ¼ cup water

Directions:

⇒ In a blender, combine all the ingredients and pulse well.
Divide into glasses and serve.

Nutrition: calories 59, fat 0,5, fiber 4,7, carbs 13,7, protein 1,9

6) Parsley Banana Smoothie

Preparation Time: 5 minutes   Cooking Time: Servings:6

Ingredients:

- 1 bunch parsley, roughly chopped
- 1 small avocado, pitted and peeled
- 2 pears, peeled and chopped
- 1 green apple, chopped

- 6 bananas, peeled and roughly chopped
- 1 cup ice
- 1 cup water

Directions:

⇒ In a blender, combine all the ingredients and pulse well.
Divide into glasses and serve for breakfast.

Nutrition: calories 234, fat 1,5, fiber 8.4, carbs 45,7, protein 2,3

7) Coconut Smoothie

Preparation Time: 5 minutes   Cooking Time: Servings:2

Ingredients:

- 1 cup ice
- 2 peaches, peeled and chopped

- 1 teaspoon lemon zest, grated
- 1 cup cold coconut milk

Directions:

⇒ In a blender, combine all the ingredients and pulse well.
Divide into glasses and serve.

Nutrition: calories 336, fat 29, fiber 5, carbs 20,9, protein 4,2

8) Walnut and Hemp Bowls

Preparation Time: 5 minutes   Cooking Time: 50 minutes   Servings:6

Ingredients:

- 2 teaspoons cinnamon powder
- 1 and ½ cups coconut flour
- 2 teaspoons nutmeg, ground
- ½ cup coconut flakes, unsweetened

- 2 teaspoons vanilla extract
- ½ cup walnuts, chopped
- 1/3 cup coconut oil, melted
- ¼ cup hemp hearts

Directions:

⇒ Spread all the ingredients out onto a lined baking sheet, toss to combine, and bake at 300 degrees F for 50 minutes, stirring every 10 minutes.

⇒ Divide into bowls and serve for breakfast.

Nutrition: calories 403, fat 28,6, fiber 17,4, carbs 28,5, protein 10,9

9) Almond Berry Bowls

Preparation Time: 5 minutes   **Cooking Time: 0 minutes**   Servings:2

Ingredients:

- 2 tablespoons pumpkin seeds
- 2 tablespoons almonds, chopped
- 1 tablespoon chia seeds
- A handful blueberries
- 1 cup almond milk

Directions:

⇒ Divide the almond milk into 2 bowls, then divide the seeds, almonds and blueberries, toss to combine and serve.

Nutrition: calories 400, fat 37,1, fiber 6,2, carbs 16,4, protein 7,2

10) Coconut Orange Bowls

Preparation Time: 5 minutes   **Cooking Time: 0 minutes**   Servings:2

Ingredients:

- 2 cups coconut milk
- ½ cup chia seeds
- Juice of ¼ lemon
- Zest from 1 orange, grated
- 1 tablespoon vanilla extract

Directions:

⇒ In a large bowl, combine all the ingredients and toss.   ⇒ Divide into 2 bowls and serve.

Nutrition: calories 672, fat 61,8, fiber 10,3, carbs 27,4, protein 8

11) Maple Coconut Bowls

Preparation Time: 10 minutes   **Cooking Time: 35 minutes**   Servings:4

Ingredients:

- 3 cups coconut flakes, unsweetened
- 1 and ½ cups almonds, chopped
- ½ cup sesame seeds
- ½ cup sunflower seeds
- ½ teaspoon cinnamon powder
- 2 tablespoons chia seeds
- 1 teaspoon vanilla extract
- 2 tablespoons coconut oil, melted

Directions:

⇒ In a bowl, mix almonds with sunflower seeds, sesame seeds, coconut, chia seeds and the cinnamon and stir.

⇒ Heat up a pot over medium heat, add the oil, vanilla and whisk, cook for about 1 minute and pour over the seeds and coconut mixture.

⇒ Stir everything, spread on a lined baking sheet, bake at 300 degrees F for 25 minutes, stirring the mixture after 15 minutes.

⇒ Divide the granola into bowls and serve.

Nutrition: calories 615, fat 47,1, fiber 10,8, carbs 45, protein 9,8

12) Beef and Chili Rolls

Preparation Time: 10 minutes   **Cooking Time: 15 minutes**   **Servings:2**

Ingredients:

- 0,5 oz green chilies, chopped
- 1 small yellow onion, chopped
- 4 eggs, egg yolks and whites separated
- ¼ cup cilantro, chopped
- 1 red bell pepper, finely cut into strips

- 2 tomatoes, chopped
- ½ cup beef meat, ground and browned for 10 minutes
- 1 avocado, peeled, pitted and chopped
- A drizzle of olive oil

Directions:

⇒ Heat up a pan with some olive oil over medium-high heat, add half of the egg whites after you've whisked them in a bowl, spread evenly, cook for 1 minute on each side and transfer to a plate.

⇒ Repeat the process with the rest of the egg whites and leave the egg "burritos" to one side.

⇒ Heat up the same pan over medium-high heat, add the onions, stir and sauté for 2 minutes.

⇒ Add chilies, bell pepper, tomato, meat, and cilantro, stir and cook for 5 minutes.

⇒ Add egg yolks, stir well and cook everything for 4-5 minutes more.

⇒ Divide the egg white burritos between 2 plates, divide the meat mixture, also divide the avocado, roll and serve for breakfast.

Nutrition: calories 489, fat 37,4, fiber 9,8, carbs 22,2, protein 21,3

13) Poached Eggs with Artichokes and Lemon Sauce

Preparation Time: 20 minutes   **Cooking Time: 30 minutes**   **Servings:2**

Ingredients:

- 1 egg white, whisked
- 4 eggs
- ¾ cup balsamic vinegar
- 4 ounces shallots, cooked and chopped
- 4 artichoke hearts, chopped
- A pinch of sea salt and black pepper

For the sauce:

- 1 tablespoon lemon juice
- ¾ cup ghee, softened
- 4 egg yolks
- ¼ teaspoon sweet paprika

Directions:

⇒ Put artichoke hearts in a bowl, add the vinegar, toss well to combine and leave aside for 20 minutes

⇒ In a bowl, mix the egg yolks with paprika and lemon juice and whisk.

⇒ Put some water into a saucepan and bring to a simmer over medium heat.

⇒ Put the bowl with the egg yolks over the simmering water and stir constantly.

⇒ Add melted ghee gradually, stir until the sauce thickens and take off heat.

⇒ Drain artichokes, arrange them on a lined baking sheet, brush them with the egg white, sprinkle salt, pepper and the chopped shallots on top, and bake at 375 degrees F for 20 minutes.

⇒ Heat up a saucepan with some water, bring to a simmer over medium heat, crack the 4 whole eggs into the pan, poach them for 1 minute and divide them between plates.

⇒ Add the baked artichokes on the side, drizzle the egg yolk sauce all over and serve.

Nutrition: calories 1130, fat 94,9, fiber 17,6, carbs 46,7, protein 30,6

14) Tomato and Kale Scramble

Preparation Time: 10 minutes   **Cooking Time: 10 minutes**   **Servings:1**

Ingredients:

- 2 eggs, whisked
- ¼ teaspoon rosemary, dried
- ½ cup cherry tomatoes halved
- 1 and ½ cups kale, chopped

- ½ teaspoon coconut oil, melted
- 3 tablespoons water
- 1 teaspoon balsamic vinegar
- ¼ avocado, peeled, pitted and chopped

Directions:

⇒ Heat up a pan with the oil over medium heat, add the water, kale, rosemary, and tomatoes, stir, cover and cook for 5 minutes.

⇒ Add the eggs, stir and scramble everything for 4 minutes more.

⇒ Add the vinegar, toss, transfer this to a plate, top with chopped avocado and serve.

Nutrition: calories 403, fat 21,3, fiber 15,5, carbs 26,2, protein 24

15) Scallion Muffins

Preparation Time: 10 minutes   **Cooking Time: 15 minutes**   **Servings:4**

Ingredients:

- 4 eggs
- 10 ham slices
- 4 tablespoons scallions, chopped

- A pinch of black pepper
- ½ teaspoon sweet paprika
- 1 tablespoon melted ghee

Directions:

⇒ Grease a muffin pan with the melted ghee and divide the ham slices in each muffin mold to shape your cups.

⇒ In a bowl, mix the eggs with scallions, pepper, and paprika, whisk well, divide this into the ham cups, and bake at 400 degrees F for 15 minutes.

⇒ Divide between plates and serve for breakfast.

Nutrition: calories 214, fat 14,2, fiber 1,2, carbs 3,6, protein 17,3

Chapter 3 - Soup & Stew Recipes

16) Herbed Chicken and Olives Stew

Preparation Time: 15 minutes   **Cooking Time: 2 hours**   **Servings:4**

Ingredients:

- 10 garlic cloves, peeled
- 30 black olives, pitted
- 2 pounds chicken breasts, skinless, boneless and cubed
- 2 cups chicken stock
- 25 ounces tomatoes, peeled, chopped

- 2 tablespoon rosemary, chopped
- 2 tablespoons parsley, chopped
- 2 tablespoons basil, chopped
- A pinch of sea salt and black pepper
- A drizzle of extra virgin olive oil

Directions:

⇒ Heat up a large saucepan with a drizzle of olive oil over medium-high heat, add the chicken, salt and pepper, and cook for 4 minutes.

⇒ Add garlic, stir and brown for 2 minutes more.

⇒ Add chicken stock, tomatoes, olives, thyme, and rosemary, stir, cover saucepan and bake in the oven at 325 degrees F for 1 hour.

⇒ Add parsley and basil, stir, bake for 45 more minutes, divide into bowls and serve.

Nutrition: calories 553, fat 24,8, fiber 4,1, carbs 13, protein 68,5

17) Leeks Oxtail and Tomato Stew

Preparation Time: 15 minutes   **Cooking Time: 6 hours**   **Servings:8**

Ingredients:

- 4 and ½ pounds oxtail, cut into medium chunks
- 2 tablespoons extra virgin olive oil
- 2 leeks, chopped
- 4 carrots, chopped
- 2 celery sticks, chopped
- 4 thyme springs, chopped
- 4 rosemary springs, chopped

- 4 cloves
- 4 bay leaves
- Black pepper to taste
- 2 tablespoons coconut flour
- 25 ounces plum tomatoes, peeled, chopped
- 1-quart beef stock

Directions:

⇒ In a roasting pan, mix oxtail with black pepper and half of the oil, toss and bake at 425 degrees F for 20 minutes.

⇒ Heat up a large saucepan with the rest of the oil over medium heat, add leeks, celery, and carrots, stir and cook for 4 minutes.

⇒ Add thyme, rosemary and bay leaves, stir and cook everything for 20 minutes.

⇒ Add flour and cloves to veggies and stir.

⇒ Also add tomatoes, the oxtail, its cooking juices and stock, stir, increase heat to high, bring to a boil, place the pot in the oven and bake at 325 degrees F for 5 hours.

⇒ Take the oxtail out of the pot, discard bones, return it to the pot, toss, divide the stew into bowls and serve.

Nutrition: calories 580, fat 32,6, fiber 3,1, carbs 12,8, protein 59,7

18) Cayenne Tomato and Eggplant Stew

Preparation Time: 10 minutes   **Cooking Time: 30 minutes**   **Servings:3**

Ingredients:

- 1 eggplant, chopped
- 1 yellow onion, chopped
- 2 tomatoes, chopped
- 1 teaspoon cumin powder

- A pinch of sea salt and black pepper
- 1 cup tomato puree
- A pinch of cayenne pepper
- ½ cup water

Directions:

⇒ Heat up a saucepan over medium-high heat, add the water, tomato paste, salt, pepper, cayenne and cumin and stir well.

⇒ Add the eggplant, tomato, and onion, stir, bring to a boil, reduce heat to medium, cook for 30 minutes, divide into bowls and serve.

Nutrition: calories 102, fat 0,8, fiber 8,8, carbs 23,4, protein 4,1

19) Nutmeg Coconut and Squash Cream

Preparation Time: 10 minutes   **Cooking Time: 50 minutes**   **Servings:4**

Ingredients:

- 1 butternut squash, halved lengthwise and deseeded
- 14 ounces coconut milk
- A pinch of sea salt and black pepper
- A handful parsley, chopped
- A pinch of nutmeg, ground

Directions:

⇒ Arrange the butternut squash halves on a lined baking sheet, place in the oven at 350 degrees F, bake for 45 minutes, cool down, scoop the flesh and transfer it to a large saucepan.

⇒ Add half of the coconut milk, blend using an immersion blender and then heat everything up over medium-low heat.

⇒ Add the rest of the coconut milk, salt, black pepper, nutmeg and parsley, blend using your immersion blender for a few seconds, cook for about 4 minutes, ladle into bowls and serve.

Nutrition: calories 245, fat 23,7, fiber 3, carbs 9,8, protein 2,7

20) Lemon Broccoli and Pesto Soup

Preparation Time: 10 minutes   **Cooking Time: 20 minutes**   **Servings:4**

Ingredients:

- 1 yellow onion, chopped
- 2 tablespoons olive oil
- 1 celery stick, chopped
- Zest of ½ lemon, grated
- 1-quart veggie stock
- 17 ounces water
- 1 teaspoon cumin, ground
- 1 broccoli head, florets separated
- 3 garlic cloves, minced
- 2 bay leaves
- Juice of ½ lemon
- A pinch of sea salt and black pepper

For the pesto:
- ½ cup almonds, chopped
- 1 garlic clove
- 2 tablespoons lemon juice
- 2 tablespoons olive oil
- 4 tablespoons green olives, pitted and chopped

Directions:

⇒ Heat up a large saucepan with 2 tablespoons olive oil over medium-high heat, add onion, lemon zest and a pinch of salt, stir and cook for 3 minutes.

⇒ Add celery and 3 garlic cloves, stir and cook for 1 minute more.

⇒ Add stock, cumin, water, and black pepper, stir, cover, bring to a boil and simmer for 10 minutes.

⇒ Add bay leaves and broccoli, stir, cover again and cook for 6 minutes more.

⇒ Take soup off the heat, discard bay leaves, transfer to a blender and pulse well. Add juice from ½ lemon, pulse again, return to the pot and heat up again over medium-low heat.

⇒ Meanwhile, in a food processor, blend the almonds with 1 garlic clove, 2 tablespoon lemon juice, 2 tablespoons olive oil and the green olives. Ladle the soup into bowls, top with the pesto you've just made and serve hot.

Nutrition: calories 201, fat 16,8, fiber 4,8, carbs 14,6, protein 5,4

21) Tomato and Peppers Soup

Preparation Time: 10 minutes   **Cooking Time: 0 minutes**   **Servings:4**

Ingredients:

- 8 tomatoes
- 1 red onion, chopped
- 1 cucumber, peeled and chopped
- 1 red bell pepper, chopped
- 1 green bell pepper, chopped
- 1 red chili pepper, chopped
- 3 garlic cloves

- 1 cup tomato juice
- 1 cup water
- 2 tablespoon apple cider vinegar
- Zest of ½ orange, grated
- ¾ cup olive oil
- A pinch of sea salt and black pepper

Directions:

⇒ In a blender, combine all the ingredients and pulse them well.

⇒ Divide the gazpacho into bowls and serve it cold.

Nutrition: calories 417, fat 38,5, fiber 5,2, carbs 21, protein 3,9

22) Mushrooms and Kale Soup

Preparation Time: 10 minutes   **Cooking Time: 15 minutes**   **Servings:4**

Ingredients:

- 1 yellow onion, chopped
- 2 carrots, chopped
- 6 mushrooms, chopped
- 1 red chili pepper, chopped
- 2 celery sticks, chopped
- 1 tablespoon coconut oil
- A pinch of sea salt and black pepper

- 4 garlic cloves, minced
- 4 ounces kale, chopped
- 15 oz fresh tomatoes, peeled, chopped
- 1 zucchini, chopped
- 1-quart veggie stock
- 1 bay leaf
- A handful parsley, chopped for serving

Directions:

⇒ Set your instant pot on Sauté mode, add oil and heat it up.

⇒ Add celery, carrots, onion, a pinch of salt and black pepper, stir and cook for 2 minutes.

⇒ Add chili pepper, garlic and the mushrooms, stir and cook for 2 minutes.

⇒ Add tomatoes, stock, bay leaf, kale and zucchinis, stir, cover pot and cook on High for 10 minutes.

⇒ Release pressure, stir soup again, discard the bay leaf, ladle into bowls, sprinkle the parsley on top and serve.

Nutrition: calories 109, fat 3,9, fiber 4,3, carbs 16,9, protein 4,1

23) Chicken, Tomato and Kale Soup

Preparation Time: 10 minutes   **Cooking Time: 15 minutes**   **Servings:2**

Ingredients:

- 1 red bell pepper, chopped
- 1 teaspoon coconut oil
- 1 yellow onion, chopped
- ¼ cup jalapeno peppers, chopped
- 2 garlic cloves, minced
- 1 tablespoon ghee, melted
- 1 teaspoon cumin, ground
- 1 teaspoon coriander, ground
- 1 teaspoon oregano, dried
- 1 and ½ cups chicken breast, skinless, boneless, cooked and shredded
- 2 and ½ cups chicken stock

- 2 cups kale, torn
- Zest of 1 lime, grated
- Juice of 1 lime
- A pinch of sea salt and black pepper
- 15 ounces fresh tomatoes, peeled, chopped
- 2 tablespoons spring onions, chopped
- 3 tablespoons pumpkin seeds, toasted
- 1 avocado, peeled, pitted and sliced
- 1 teaspoon sweet paprika
- 3 tablespoons coriander, chopped

Directions:

⇒ Heat up a large saucepan with the oil over medium heat, add the onion, stir and sauté for 2 minutes.

⇒ Add red bell peppers, the garlic, jalapenos, oregano, cumin, coriander, and ghee, stir and cook for 1 minute more.

⇒ Add tomatoes, kale, chicken, lime zest, stock, lime juice, salt and pepper, stir, bring to a boil, cook for 5 minutes and take off the heat.

⇒ Ladle the soup into bowls, top with pumpkin seeds, green onion, paprika, chopped coriander and avocado and serve.

Nutrition: calories 1227, fat 53,2, fiber 14,2, carbs 60,7, protein 127,6

24) Broccoli and Spinach Soup

Preparation Time: 10 minutes   **Cooking Time: 25 minutes**   **Servings:6**

Ingredients:

- 2 leeks, chopped
- 2 tablespoons ghee
- 4 celery sticks, chopped
- 4 garlic cloves, minced
- 2 broccoli heads, florets separated
- 1 small cauliflower head, florets separated

- 2 handfuls spinach, chopped
- 8 cups veggie stock
- 1 handful parsley, chopped
- 1 tablespoon coconut cream
- A pinch of nutmeg, ground
- Black pepper to taste

Directions:

⇒ Heat up a large saucepan with the ghee over medium heat, add garlic and leeks, stir and cook for 3 minutes.

⇒ Add the broccoli, celery and cauliflower, stir and cook for 5 minutes,

⇒ Add stock, bring to a boil, cover saucepan and cook for 15 minutes.

⇒ Add parsley, spinach, black pepper and the nutmeg, stir and blend using an immersion blender.

⇒ Ladle soup into bowls and serve with the coconut cream on top.

Nutrition: calories 120, fat 8, fiber 4,4, carbs 16, protein 4

25) Mustard Mushroom Cream

Preparation Time: 10 minutes   **Cooking Time: 20 minutes**   **Servings:4**

Ingredients:

- 1 ounce dried porcini mushrooms
- 1 leek, chopped
- 2 tablespoons olive oil
- 1 celery stick, chopped
- 3 garlic cloves, chopped
- 14 brown mushrooms, chopped
- 1 tablespoon thyme, chopped
- 3 cups veggie stock

- 1 sweet potato, peeled and chopped
- 2 bay leaves
- ½ teaspoon Dijon mustard
- 1 teaspoon lemon zest, grated
- ½ teaspoon black pepper
- 1 tablespoon lemon juice
- 3 tablespoons coconut butter

Directions:

⇒ Put dried mushrooms in a bowl, cover them with boiling water, leave aside for 10 minutes, strain, reserve water and chop them.

⇒ Heat up a large saucepan with the oil over medium heat, add celery and leek, stir and cook for 5 minutes.

⇒ Add mushrooms, thyme, garlic and sweet potatoes, stir and cook for 1 minute.

⇒ Add dried mushrooms and half of their liquid, stock, bay leaves, mustard, black pepper and lemon zest, stir, cover pan and simmer soup over medium heat for 15 minutes.

⇒ Discard bay leaves, use an immersion blender to make your mushroom cream, add lemon juice and the coconut butter, stir well, ladle into bowls and serve.

Nutrition: calories 171, fat 8,8, fiber 4,2, carbs 18,9, protein 4,8

26) Garlic Cod Soup

Preparation Time: 2 hours and 10 minutes   **Cooking Time: 30 minutes**   **Servings:4**

Ingredients:

- 1 pound cod fillets, skinless, boneless and cubed
- 10 garlic cloves, minced
- 3 tablespoons olive oil
- 1 tablespoon lemon juice
- ¼ cup parsley, chopped
- 1 yellow onion, chopped
- 2 tomatoes, chopped

- 1 tablespoon tomato paste
- 2 bay leaves
- 2 and ½ cups water
- A pinch of sea salt and black pepper
- 1 pound shrimp, peeled and deveined
- 10 cherry tomatoes, halved
- 1 pound mussels, scrubbed

Directions:

⇒ In a bowl, mix 6 garlic cloves with 2 tablespoons oil, parsley, lemon juice and the fish, toss, cover the bowl and keep in the fridge for 2 hours.

⇒ Heat up a large saucepan with the rest of the oil over medium-high heat, add the onion, stir and cook for 2 minutes.

⇒ Add the rest of the garlic, the tomatoes, tomato paste, bay leaves, water, salt, pepper and the fish, stir, bring to a simmer and cook for 10 minutes.

⇒ Add shrimp, cherry tomatoes and mussels, stir, cook for 6 minutes more, ladle into bowls and serve.

Nutrition: calories 508, fat 17, fiber 2,3, carbs 16, protein 71,1

27) Coconut Shrimp Soup

Preparation Time: 10 minutes   **Cooking Time: 30 minutes**   **Servings:4**

Ingredients:

- 5 tablespoons curry paste
- 1 tablespoon coconut oil, melted
- 1 big chicken breast, skinless, boneless and cut into thin strips
- 4 tablespoons coconut aminos
- 2 cups chicken stock
- Juice of 1 lime
- 1 and ½ cups coconut milk
- 1 pound shrimp, peeled and deveined

- ½ cup coconut cream
- A small broccoli head, florets separated
- 5 Chinese broccoli leaves, chopped
- 1 zucchini, chopped
- 1 carrot, chopped
- 1 cucumber, chopped
- 1 tablespoon cilantro, chopped for serving

Directions:

⇒ Heat up a large saucepan with the oil over medium heat, add curry paste, stir and heat up for 1 minute.

⇒ Add the chicken, stir and cook for 1 minute more.

⇒ Add stock and lime juice, stir and cook for 2 minutes.

⇒ Add coconut cream, aminos and coconut milk, stir and cook for 10 minutes.

⇒ Add broccoli leaves, broccoli florets and carrots, stir and cook for 3 minutes.

⇒ Add shrimp and zucchini, stir and cook for 2 minutes.

⇒ Ladle into bowls, top with cilantro and cucumber and serve.

Nutrition: calories 1252, fat 98,5, fiber 11,2, carbs 40,8, protein 62,3

28) Coconut Zucchini Cream

Preparation Time: 10 minutes   **Cooking Time: 20 minutes**   **Servings:4**

Ingredients:

- 1 onion, chopped
- 3 zucchinis, cut into medium chunks
- 2 tablespoons coconut milk
- 2 garlic cloves, minced

- 4 cups chicken stock
- 2 tablespoons coconut oil
- A pinch of sea salt and black pepper

Directions:

⇒ Heat up a large saucepan with the oil over medium heat, add zucchinis, garlic, and onion, stir and cook for 5 minutes.

⇒ Add stock, salt, pepper, stir, bring to a boil, cover pan, simmer soup for 20 minutes and take off heat.

⇒ Add coconut milk, blend using an immersion blender, ladle into bowls and serve.

Nutrition: calories 122, fat 9,5, fiber 2,4, carbs 9,1, protein 3

29) Curry Coconut Soup

Preparation Time: 10 minutes   **Cooking Time: 15 minutes**   **Servings:2**

Ingredients:

- 1 brown onion, chopped
- 1 tablespoon coconut oil
- 2 zucchinis, cubed
- A pinch of sea salt and black pepper
- 2 teaspoons turmeric powder
- 3 garlic cloves, chopped

- 1 teaspoon curry powder
- 1 cup coconut milk
- 1 cup veggie stock
- 2 tablespoons lime juice
- 1 tablespoon cilantro, chopped

Directions:

⇒ Heat up a large saucepan with the oil over medium heat, add onion, stir and sauté for 4 minutes.

⇒ Add garlic, salt, pepper, and zucchinis, stir and cook for 1 minute.

⇒ Add turmeric and curry powder, stir well and cook for 1 minute more.

⇒ Add coconut milk and stock, stir, bring to a boil, cover pan and simmer soup for 10 minutes.

⇒ Add lime juice and cilantro, stir, ladle into bowls and serve.

Nutrition: calories 414, fat 32,4, fiber 6,9, carbs 23,8, protein 6,4

30) Shallot and Cauliflower Cream

Preparation Time: 10 minutes   **Cooking Time: 20 minutes**   **Servings:2**

Ingredients:

- 1 yellow onion, chopped
- 2 tablespoons olive oil
- 1 cauliflower head, florets separated and chopped
- 3 cups veggie stock
- 3 garlic cloves, minced

- A pinch of sea salt and black pepper
- ¾ cup shallots, cooked and chopped
- 1 teaspoon coconut oil, melted
- 1 egg
- 2 tablespoons cilantro, chopped

Directions:

⇒ Heat up a large saucepan with the olive oil over medium heat, add the onion, stir and sauté for 4 minutes.

⇒ Add stock, cauliflower and garlic, stir, bring to a boil, reduce heat to medium-low, season with salt and black pepper, cover the saucepan and simmer soup for 10 minutes.

⇒ Meanwhile, put water in a pot, bring to a boil, place a bowl on top of boiling water, crack the egg into the bowl, whisk it for 3 minutes and take off the heat.

⇒ Blend the soup using an immersion blender, add whisked egg and blend again.

⇒ Ladle into bowls, sprinkle crumbled shallots and cilantro on top and serve.

Nutrition: calories 291, fat 21,7, fiber 4,6, carbs 26,9, protein 7,8

31) Sweet Potato and Nettle Cream

Preparation Time: 10 minutes　　　**Cooking Time: 20 minutes**　　　**Servings:3**

Ingredients:

- 1 tablespoon coconut oil, melted
- 1 cup sweet potato, chopped
- 1 yellow onion, chopped
- ½ broccoli head, florets separated
- ½ cauliflower head, florets separated
- 3 garlic cloves, minced
- Zest of 1 lemon, grated
- 1 teaspoon Dijon mustard

- 3 and ½ cups veggie stock
- A pinch of sea salt and black pepper
- 4 cups nettles
- Juice of 1 lemon
- 5 thyme springs, leaves separated
- 2 small shallots, cooked and crumbled
- ½ cup coconut cream

Directions:

⇒ Heat up a large saucepan with the coconut oil over medium heat, add sweet potato, onion, broccoli, and cauliflower, stir and cook for 6 minutes.

⇒ Add the garlic, veggie stock, lemon zest, salt, pepper, and mustard, stir, bring to a boil, reduce the heat and simmer the soup for 10 minutes

⇒ Meanwhile, put some water in a pot, bring to a boil, cut nettles leaves with scissors, add the leaves to the boiling water, cook them for 2 minutes, drain and transfer them to the saucepan with the soup.

⇒ Cook for 3 minutes more, add lemon juice, blend everything using an immersion blender and then heat up the soup again.

⇒ Add thyme and coconut cream, stir, cook for 1 minute and ladle into soup bowls.

⇒ Top with the shallots and serve.

Nutrition:　　　calories 766, fat 44,7, fiber 25,1, carbs 90,7, protein 16,1

32) Garlic Potato and Pine Nuts Cream

Preparation Time: 10 minutes　　　**Cooking Time: 20 minutes**　　　**Servings:2**

Ingredients:

- 4 tablespoons olive oil
- 5 garlic cloves, minced
- 1 sweet potato, chopped
- ½ teaspoon cumin seeds

- 14 ounces veggie stock
- A pinch of sea salt and black pepper
- 4 tablespoons pine nuts, toasted

Directions:

⇒ Heat up a large saucepan with the oil over medium heat, add the garlic, stir and cook for 4 minutes.

⇒ Add the sweet potato, stock, cumin, salt and black pepper, stir, bring to a boil and cook for 15 minutes.

⇒ Blend the soup using an immersion blender and mix with half of the pine nuts.

⇒ Blend again, ladle into bowls and sprinkle the rest of the pine nuts on top.

Nutrition:　　　calories 445, fat 45, fiber 2,8, carbs 21,8, protein 4,1

Chapter 4 -   Side Recipes

33) Asparagus and Green Onions Mix

Preparation Time: 10 minutes   **Cooking Time: 10 minutes**   **Servings:4**

Ingredients:

- 1 pound asparagus, trimmed
- A pinch of sea salt and black pepper
- 8 green onions, thinly sliced
- 2 tablespoons coconut oil

- 2 tablespoons balsamic vinegar
- 2 tablespoons walnuts, chopped
- 1 pound mushrooms, chopped

Directions:

⇒ In a bowl, mix the vinegar with salt, pepper and half of the oil and whisk.

⇒ Put some water in a large saucepan, bring to a boil over medium heat, add asparagus, cook for 3 minutes, drain and transfer to a bowl filled with cold water.

⇒ Heat up a pan with the rest of the oil over medium-high heat, add mushrooms and cook them for 4-5 minutes stirring from time to time.

⇒ Add onions, stir and cook for 1 minute.

⇒ Add drained asparagus, stir, cook 3 more minutes and take off heat.

⇒ Add vinegar mix, stir and divide between plates.

⇒ Sprinkle the walnuts at the end and serve as a side dish!

Nutrition: calories 141, fat 9,6, fiber 4,6, carbs 10,8, protein 7,5

34) Baked Mushrooms

Preparation Time: 10 minutes   **Cooking Time: 25 minutes**   **Servings:4**

Ingredients:

- 4 garlic cloves, minced
- 2 tablespoons extra virgin olive oil

- 16 ounces mushrooms, sliced
- A pinch of sea salt and black pepper

Directions:

⇒ In a baking dish, combine all the ingredients, toss, and bake at 375 degrees F for 25 minutes.

⇒ Divide everything between plates and serve as a side dish.

Nutrition: calories 89, fat 7,3, fiber 1,2, carbs 4,7, protein 3,8

35) Garlic and Basil Tomatoes

Preparation Time: 5 minutes   **Cooking Time: 20 minutes**   **Servings:4**

Ingredients:

- 2 tablespoons extra virgin olive oil
- 20 ounces colored cherry tomatoes, halved
- 6 garlic cloves, finely minced

- A pinch of sea salt and black pepper
- 1 tablespoon basil leaves, finely chopped

Directions:

⇒ In a baking dish, combine all the ingredients, place in the oven at 375 degrees F and bake for 20 minutes.

⇒ Divide between plates and serve as a side dish.

Nutrition: calories 91, fat 7,4, fiber 1,9, carbs 6,8, protein 2,1

36) Garlic Spinach

Preparation Time: 10 minutes **Cooking Time: 33 minutes** **Servings:3**

Ingredients:

- 3 cups spinach, torn
- 3 yellow onions, sliced
- 3 garlic cloves, finely minced
- A pinch of sea salt and black pepper

- 10 mushrooms, sliced
- 1 tablespoon coconut oil, melted
- 1 tablespoon balsamic vinegar
- 1 tablespoon ghee

Directions:

⇒ Heat up a pan with the oil and ghee over medium-high heat, add garlic and onions, stir and cook for 10 minutes.

⇒ Reduce temperature to low and cook onions for 20 minutes, stirring from time to time.

⇒ Add vinegar, mushrooms, salt and pepper, stir and cook for 10 minutes.

⇒ Add spinach, stir, cook for 3 minutes more, take off heat, divide between plates and serve as a side dish.

Nutrition: calories 146, fat 9,2, fiber 3,7, carbs 14,4, protein 4,2

37) Parsley Carrot Mash

Preparation Time: 6 minutes **Cooking Time: 20 minutes** **Servings:4**

Ingredients:

- 1 pound rutabaga, peeled and chopped
- A pinch of sea salt and black pepper
- 4 tablespoons ghee

- 1 pound carrots, chopped
- 1 tablespoon parsley, chopped

Directions:

⇒ Put rutabaga and carrots in a pot, add water to cover, place on stove, bring to a boil over medium heat and cook for 20 minutes.

⇒ Drain carrots and rutabaga, transfer them to a bowl, mash with a potato masher, mix with ghee, salt and pepper, stir well, divide between plates, sprinkle parsley on top and serve as a side dish.

Nutrition: calories 200, fat 13, fiber 5,7, carbs 12,4, protein 2,4

38) Balsamic Peppers and Capers Mix

Preparation Time: 10 minutes **Cooking Time: 1 hour** **Servings:4**

Ingredients:

- 6 bell peppers (green, yellow and red)
- 1 garlic clove, finely minced
- 2 tablespoon capers
- 2 tablespoons extra virgin olive oil

- ¼ cup balsamic vinegar
- A pinch of sea salt and black pepper
- 2 tablespoons parsley, finely chopped

Directions:

⇒ Arrange bell peppers on a lined baking sheet, place them in the oven at 400 degrees F and bake for 40 minutes.

⇒ Transfer bell peppers to a bowl, cover and leave them aside for 10 minutes.

⇒ Peel the peppers, discard seeds, cut into strips and transfer them to a bowl.

⇒ Add sea salt and pepper, vinegar, oil, garlic, capers and parsley, toss to coat, divide between plates and serve as a side dish.

Nutrition: calories 123, fat 7,5, fiber 2,6, carbs 14,2, protein 2

39) Herbed Potatoes

Preparation Time: 10 minutes   **Cooking Time: 25 minutes**   **Servings:3**

Ingredients:

- 2 pounds sweet potatoes, cut into wedges
- A pinch of sea salt and black pepper
- ¼ cup ghee, melted
- 3 teaspoons thyme and rosemary, dried

Directions:

⇒ In a bowl, mix potato wedges with ghee, salt, pepper and dried herbs and toss to coat.

⇒ Spread potatoes on a lined baking sheet and bake in the oven at 425 degrees F for 25 minutes.

⇒ Divide between plates and serve as a side dish.

Nutrition: calories 512, fat 7,7, fiber 13,1, carbs 85,6, protein 4,9

40) Lemon Chili Cabbage

Preparation Time: 10 minutes   **Cooking Time: 30 minutes**   **Servings:4**

Ingredients:

- 1 green cabbage head, cut into medium wedges
- A pinch of sea salt and black pepper
- A pinch of red chili flakes
- A pinch of garlic powder
- 2 tablespoons extra virgin olive oil
- Juice of 2 lemons

Directions:

⇒ Brush the cabbage with olive oil, salt and pepper, sprinkle garlic powder and pepper flakes, arrange it on a lined baking sheet and bake at 450 degrees F for 30 minutes, flipping the cabbage wedges halfway.

⇒ Divide between plates, drizzle the lemon juice on top and serve.

Nutrition: calories 118, fat 7,3, fiber 4,8, carbs 14, protein 2,7

41) Paprika Okra Mix

Preparation Time: 10 minutes   **Cooking Time: 25 minutes**   **Servings:3**

Ingredients:

- 18 okra pods, sliced
- A pinch of sea salt and black pepper
- 1 teaspoon sweet paprika
- 1 tablespoon extra-virgin olive oil

Directions:

⇒ Combine all the ingredients in a baking dish, place in the oven and bake at 425 degrees F for 15 minutes.

⇒ Divide between plates and serve as a side dish.

Nutrition: calories 107, fat 5, fiber 5,3, carbs 12,4, protein 3,2

Chapter 5 -   Snack & Appetizer Recipes

42) Hot Artichoke Bowls

Preparation Time: 10 minutes   **Cooking Time: 0 minutes**   Servings:4

Ingredients:

- 1 big romaine lettuce head, chopped
- ½ cup artichoke hearts, chopped
- ½ cup hot peppers, chopped
- ½ cup black olives, pitted and chopped
- For the dressing:
- 1 tablespoon parsley, chopped

- 1 garlic clove, minced
- 1 teaspoon oregano, dried
- Black pepper to taste
- A pinch of sea salt
- ¾ cup avocado oil
- ¼ cup red wine vinegar

Directions:

⇒ In a bowl, combine all the ingredients, toss, divide into small cups and serve as an appetizer.

Nutrition: calories 109, fat 7,2, fiber 5, carbs 10,2, protein 3

43) Banana and Walnut Snack

Preparation Time: 5 minutes   **Cooking Time: 1 hour and 30 minutes**   Servings:6

Ingredients:

- 2 and ¼ cup walnuts, chopped
- 1/3 cup coconut sugar
- 5 tablespoons coconut oil

- 1 cup coconut flakes, unsweetened
- 1 teaspoon vanilla extract
- 2 cups banana slices, dried

Directions:

⇒ In a crock pot, combine all the ingredients, cover and cook on Low for 1 hour and 30 minutes.

⇒ Divide everything into bowls and serve as a snack.

Nutrition: calories 464, fat 29, fiber 7,8, carbs 56,5, protein 5,3

44) Squash Wraps

Preparation Time: 10 minutes   **Cooking Time: 40 minutes**   Servings:4

Ingredients:

- 10 ounces turkey meat, cooked, sliced
- 2 pounds butternut squash, cubed
- 1 teaspoon chili powder

- 1 teaspoon garlic powder
- 1 teaspoon sweet paprika
- Black pepper to taste

Directions:

⇒ In a bowl, mix butternut squash cubes with chili powder, black pepper, garlic powder and paprika and toss to coat.

⇒ Wrap squash pieces in turkey slices, place them all on a lined baking sheet, place in the oven at 350 degrees F, bake for 20 minutes, flip and bake for 20 minutes more.

⇒ Arrange squash bites on a platter and serve.

Nutrition: calories 223, fat 3,8, fiber 4,5, carbs 26,5, protein 23

45) Thyme Zucchini Fries

Preparation Time: 10 minutes   **Cooking Time: 12 minutes**   **Servings:4**

Ingredients:

- 1 zucchini, thinly sliced
- A pinch of sea salt
- Black pepper to taste
- 1 teaspoon thyme, dried

- 1 egg
- 1 teaspoon garlic powder
- 1 cup almond flour

Directions:

⇒ In a bowl, whisk the egg with a pinch of salt.

⇒ Put the flour in another bowl and mix it with thyme, black pepper, and garlic powder.

⇒ Dredge zucchini slices in the egg mix and then in flour.

⇒ Arrange chips on a lined baking sheet, place in the oven at 450 degrees F and bake for 6 minutes on each side,

⇒ Serve the zucchini chips as a snack.

Nutrition: calories 106, fat 8,2, fiber 2,1, carbs 5,2, protein 5,1

46) Cheese Bites

Preparation Time: 5 minutes   **Cooking Time: 10 minutes**   **Servings: 24 pieces**

Ingredients:

- 1/3 cup tomatoes, chopped
- ½ cup bell peppers, mixed and chopped
- ½ cup tomato sauce

- 4 ounces almond cheese, cubed
- 2 tablespoons basil, chopped
- Black pepper to taste

Directions:

⇒ Divide tomato and bell pepper pieces into a muffin tray.

⇒ Also divide the tomato sauce, basil and almond cheese cubes, sprinkle black pepper at the end, place cups in the oven at 400 degrees F and bake for 10 minutes.

⇒ Arrange the meal on a platter and serve.

Nutrition: calories 59, fat 4,5, fiber 0,1, carbs 2, protein 2,5

47) Turkey Balls

Preparation Time: 10 minutes   **Cooking Time: 40 minutes**   **Servings:20**

Ingredients:

- 1 pound turkey meat, ground
- 1 tablespoon coconut oil, melted
- 1 yellow onion, chopped
- 1 egg
- 1 cup coconut flour

- 1 teaspoon Italian seasoning
- A pinch of sea salt
- Black pepper to taste
- 2 tablespoons parsley, chopped

Directions:

⇒ In a bowl, mix turkey meat with half of the flour, a pinch of salt, black pepper, Italian seasoning, parsley, onion, egg and hot sauce and stir well.

⇒ Put the rest of the flour in another bowl.

⇒ Shape 20 turkey meatballs and dip each one in flour.

⇒ Heat up a pan with the oil over medium-high heat, add meatballs, cook them for 4 minutes on each side, transfer to paper towels to remove any excess grease, place all of them on a platter and serve.

Nutrition: calories 71, fat 2,6, fiber 2,2, carbs 4,1, protein 7,7

48) Coconut Chicken Bites

Preparation Time: 10 minutes **Cooking Time: 20 minutes** **Servings:4**

Ingredients:

- 1 pound chicken tenders
- 1 egg, whisked
- A pinch of sea salt

- 1/3 cup coconut, unsweetened and shredded
- ¼ cup coconut flour

Directions:

⇒ In a bowl, mix coconut with coconut flour and a pinch of sea salt and stir.

⇒ Put whisked egg in another bowl.

⇒ Dip chicken pieces in egg, then in coconut mixture, arrange them all on a lined baking sheet and bake at 350 degrees F for 25 minutes.

⇒ Serve as a snack.

Nutrition: calories 330, fat 13,6, fiber 8,1, carbs 13,6, protein 36,9

49) Dehydrated Beef Bites

Preparation Time: 6 hours **Cooking Time: 6 hours** **Servings:6**

Ingredients:

- ½ cup coconut aminos
- 2 and ½ pounds beef, thinly sliced
- 2 tablespoons gluten free liquid smoke

- ¼ cup coconut sugar
- ¼ cup apple cider vinegar
- A pinch of sea salt

Directions:

⇒ In a bowl, mix vinegar with coconut sugar, aminos, liquid smoke, ginger and a pinch of salt and stir well.

⇒ Add meat slices, toss to coat well, cover and keep in the fridge for 6 hours.

⇒ Transfer meat slices to your preheated dehydrator at 165 degrees F and dehydrate them for 6 hours.

⇒ Transfer beef jerky to a bowl and serve as a snack.

Nutrition: calories 273, fat 8,3, fiber 0, carbs 12,9, protein 33,3

50) Chicken Platter

Preparation Time: 3 hours **Cooking Time: 15 minutes** **Servings:4**

Ingredients:

- 2 tablespoons parsley, chopped
- 4 chicken breasts, cubed

- ¾ cup garlic powder
- Black pepper to taste

Directions:

⇒ In a bowl, mix chicken with garlic powder, black pepper, and parsley, stir well, cover and keep in the fridge for 3 hours.

⇒ Arrange chicken pieces on skewers, place them all on preheated grill and cook for 15 minutes, flipping once.

⇒ Arrange skewers on a platter and serve as an appetizer.

Nutrition: calories 485, fat 22,9, fiber 2,6, carbs 18,6, protein 53,1

51) Baked Kale Bowls

Preparation Time: 10 minutes **Cooking Time: 20 minutes** **Servings:6**

Ingredients:

- 1 tablespoon avocado oil
- 1 bunch kale, leaves separated

- A pinch of sea salt
- Black pepper to taste

Directions:

⇒ Pat dry kale leaves, arrange them on a lined baking sheet, drizzle the oil, sprinkle a pinch of sea salt and black pepper to taste, place in the oven at 275 degrees F and bake for 20 minutes.

⇒ Serve the chips cold.

Nutrition: calories 9, fat 0,3, fiber 0,3, carbs 1,3, protein 0,4

52) Herbed Snack

Preparation Time: 10 minutes   **Cooking Time: 14 minutes**   **Servings:40**

Ingredients:

- ¼ cup coconut flour
- 1 cup almond flour
- ½ cup sesame seeds, toasted and ground
- 2 tablespoons tapioca flour
- A pinch of sea salt

- Black pepper to taste
- 1 teaspoon onion powder
- 1 teaspoon rosemary, chopped
- ½ teaspoon thyme, chopped
- 2 eggs
- 3 tablespoons olive oil

Directions:

⇒ In a bowl, mix sesame seeds with coconut flour, almond flour, tapioca flour, salt, pepper, rosemary, thyme and onion powder and stir well.

⇒ In another bowl, whisk eggs with the oil and stir well.

⇒ Add this to flour mix and knead until you obtain a dough.

⇒ Shape a disk out of this dough, flatten well and cut 40 crackers out of it.

⇒ Arrange them all on a lined baking sheet, place in the oven at 375 degrees F and bake for 14 minutes.

⇒ Leave your crackers to cool down and serve them as a snack.

Nutrition: calories 37, fat 2,9, fiber 1,1, carbs 2,2, protein 1,1

53) Pumpkin Crakers

Preparation Time: 10 minutes   **Cooking Time: 3 hours**   **Servings:40**

Ingredients:

- ½ cup chia seeds
- 1 cup flaxseed, ground
- ½ cup pumpkin seeds
- 1/3 cup sesame seeds
- A pinch of sea salt

- 1 and ¼ cups water
- ½ teaspoon garlic powder
- 1 teaspoon thyme, dried
- 1 teaspoon basil, dried

Directions:

⇒ Put pumpkin seeds in your food processor, pulse well and transfer them to a bowl.

⇒ Add flaxseed, sesame seeds, chia, salt, water, garlic powder, thyme and basil and stir well until they combine.

⇒ Spread this on a lined baking sheet, press well, cuts into 40 pieces, place in the oven at 200 degrees F and bake for 3 hours.

⇒ Leave your crackers to cool down before serving them as a snack.

Nutrition: calories 35, fat 2,5, fiber 1,2, carbs 1,7, protein 1,3

54) Cashew Crackers

Preparation Time: 30 minutes   **Cooking Time: 0 minutes**   **Servings:10**

Ingredients:

- 1 teaspoon vanilla extract
- 1 cup coconut flakes, unsweetened
- 2 cups cashews
- 1 and ¼ cups figs, dried

- A pinch of sea salt
- 1/3 cup cocoa butter
- ¾ cup cocoa powder
- 1 tablespoon cocoa powder

Directions:

⇒ In your food processor, mix figs with vanilla, cashews, a pinch of salt, cocoa powder and coconut and blend them well.

⇒ Transfer this into a baking dish and press well.

⇒ Put cocoa powder and cocoa butter in a heatproof bowl, place in your microwave for 3 minutes until it melts.

⇒ Pour this over coconut mix, spread well, place in your freezer for 20 minutes, cut into crackers and serve as a snack.

Nutrition: calories 1504, fat 28,1, fiber 52,2, carbs 331,5, protein 22,1

Chapter 6 -   Meat Recipes

55) Salsa Pork Mix

Preparation Time: 12 hours and 10 minutes **Cooking Time: 8 hours and 20 minutes** **Servings:4**

Ingredients:

- ½ cup paleo salsa
- ½ cup beef stock
- ½ cup enchilada sauce
- 3 pounds organic pork shoulder
- 2 green chilies, chopped
- 1 tablespoon garlic powder

- 1 tablespoon chili powder
- 1 teaspoon onion powder
- 1 teaspoon cumin, ground
- 1 teaspoon sweet paprika
- Black pepper to taste

Directions:

⇒ In a bowl, mix chili powder with onion and garlic one.

⇒ Add cumin, paprika and pepper to taste and stir everything.

⇒ Add pork, rub well and keep in the fridge for 12 hours.

⇒ Transfer pork to a slow cooker, add enchilada sauce, stock, salsa and green chilies, stir, cover and cook on Low for 8 hours.

⇒ Transfer pork to a plate, leave aside to cool down and shred.

⇒ Strain sauce from slow cooker into a pan, bring to a boil over medium heat and simmer for 8 minutes stirring all the time.

⇒ Add shredded pork to the sauce, stir, reduce heat to medium and cook for 20 more minutes.

⇒ Divide between plates and serve hot.

Nutrition: calories 1013, fat 73, carbs 4,3, fiber 1,6, protein 80,4

56) Smoked Pork Ribs

Preparation Time: 15 minutes **Cooking Time: 2 hours and 47 minutes** **Servings:4**

Ingredients:

- 1 tablespoon smoked paprika
- ½ tablespoon onion powder
- ½ tablespoon garlic powder
- ½ teaspoon cayenne pepper
- 4 pounds baby ribs
- 1 cup paleo BBQ sauce

- 4 teaspoons Sriracha
- ¼ cup cilantro, chopped
- ¼ cup chives, chopped
- ¼ cup parsley, chopped
- Black pepper to taste

Directions:

⇒ In a bowl, mix paprika with onion powder, garlic powder, pepper and cayenne and stir well.

⇒ Add ribs, toss to coat and arrange them on a lined baking sheet.

⇒ Place in the oven at 325 degrees F and bake them for 2 hours and 30 minutes.

⇒ In a bowl, mix BBQ sauce with Sriracha and stir well.

⇒ Take ribs out of the oven, mix them with BBQ sauce, place them on preheated grill over medium-high heat and cook for 7 minutes on each side.

⇒ Divide ribs between plates, sprinkle chives, cilantro, and parsley on top and serve.

Nutrition: calories 1483, fat 122,3, fiber 1,1, carbs 9,5, protein 81,8

57) Sage Pork

Preparation Time: 10 minutes   **Cooking Time: 30 minutes**   **Servings:4**

Ingredients:

- 8 sage springs
- 4 pork chops, bone-in
- 4 tablespoons ghee
- 4 garlic cloves, crushed

- 1 tablespoon coconut oil
- A pinch of sea salt
- Black pepper to taste

Directions:

⇒ Season pork chops with a pinch of sea salt and pepper to taste.

⇒ Heat up a pan with the oil over medium high heat, add pork chops and cook for 10 minutes turning them often.

⇒ Take pork chops off heat, add ghee, sage, and garlic and toss to coat.

⇒ Return to heat, cook for 4 minutes often stirring, divide between plates and serve.

Nutrition: calories 402, fat 36, fiber 0,1, carbs 1, protein 18,2

58) Balsamic Pork Mix

Preparation Time: 10 minutes   **Cooking Time: 45 minutes**   **Servings:4**

Ingredients:

- 1 yellow onion, chopped
- 1 organic pork tenderloin
- 2 pears, chopped
- 2 garlic cloves, minced
- 1 tablespoon chives, chopped
- ¼ cup walnuts, chopped

- 3 tablespoons balsamic vinegar
- Black pepper to taste
- ½ cup chicken stock
- 1 tablespoon coconut oil
- 1 tablespoon lemon juice

Directions:

⇒ In a bowl, mix walnuts with pear, chives, pepper and lemon juice and stir well.

⇒ Heat up a pan with the oil over medium-high heat, add tenderloin and brown for 3 minutes on each side.

⇒ Reduce heat, add onion and garlic, stir and cook for 2 minutes.

⇒ Add balsamic vinegar, stock, pear mix, stir, place in the oven at 400 degrees F and bake for 20 minutes.

⇒ Take pork out of the oven, leave aside for 4 minutes, slice, divide between plates and serve with pear salsa on top.

Nutrition: calories 271, fat 11,2, fiber 4,4, carbs 20,1, protein 24,6

59) Pork with Carrots and Sauce

Preparation Time: 10 minutes   **Cooking Time: 45 minutes**   **Servings:4**

Ingredients:

- 15 oz turkey mince
- A handful arugula
- Black pepper to taste
- 1 grass fed pork tenderloin
- 1 tablespoon coconut oil

  For the puree:
- 1 sweet potato, chopped
- 3 carrots, chopped
- A pinch of sea salt

- Black pepper to taste
- 1 tablespoon curry paste

  For the sauce:
- 2 tablespoons balsamic vinegar
- 1 teaspoon mustard
- 2 shallots, chopped
- Black pepper to taste
- 4 tablespoons extra virgin olive oil

Directions:

⇒ Slice pork tenderloin in half horizontally but not all the way and open it up.

⇒ Use a meat tenderizer to even it up.

⇒ Place turkey mince in the middle, roll pork around it, tie with twine, season pepper to taste and leave to one side.

⇒ Heat up an oven proof pan with the coconut oil over medium-high heat, add pork roll, cook for 3 minutes on each side, place in the oven at 350 degrees F and bake for 25 minutes.

⇒ Meanwhile, put potatoes and carrots in a large saucepan, add water to cover, bring to a boil over medium-high heat, cook for 20 minutes, drain and transfer to a food processor.

⇒ Pulse a few times until you obtain a puree, add a pinch of sea salt and pepper to taste, blend again, transfer to a bowl and leave aside.

⇒ Take pork roll out of the oven, slice and divide between plates.

⇒ Heat up a pan with the olive oil over medium-high heat, add shallots, stir and cook for 10 minutes.

⇒ Add balsamic vinegar, mustard, pepper, stir well and take off heat. Divide carrots puree next to pork slices, drizzle vinegar sauce on to and serve with arugula on the side.

Nutrition: calories 495, fat 29,5, carbs 2,2, fiber 17,5, protein 21,8

60) Garlic Pork and Strawberries

Preparation Time: 10 minutes   **Cooking Time: 35 minutes**   **Servings:4**

Ingredients:

- 4 pounds pork tenderloin
- 1 cup strawberries, sliced
- 10 thin turkey fillet strips
- A pinch of sea salt

- Black pepper to taste
- 4 garlic cloves, minced
- ½ cup balsamic vinegar
- 2 tablespoons extra virgin olive oil

Directions:

⇒ Wrap turkey strips around tenderloin, secure with toothpicks and season with salt and pepper.

⇒ Heat up your grill over indirect medium high heat, put tenderloin on it and cook for 30 minutes.

⇒ Heat up a pan with the oil over medium high heat, add garlic, stir and cook for 2 minutes.

⇒ Add vinegar and half of the strawberries, stir and bring to a boil.

⇒ Reduce heat to medium and simmer for 10 minutes.

⇒ Add black pepper to taste and the rest of the strawberries and stir.

⇒ Baste pork with some of the sauce and continue cooking over indirect heat until turkey is brown enough.

⇒ Transfer pork to a cutting board, leave aside for a few minutes to cool down, slice and divide between plates.

⇒ Serve with the strawberry sauce right away.

Nutrition: calories 981, fat 24,3, carbs 4, fiber 0,8, protein 174,1

61) Turkey with Peppers and Tomatoes

Preparation Time: 15 minutes   **Cooking Time: 45 minutes**   **Servings:6**

Ingredients:

- 20 ounces ground turkey
- 2 green bell peppers, chopped
- 3 sweet potatoes, chopped
- 1-pint grape tomatoes, chopped
- A pinch of sea salt

- Black pepper to taste
- 2 garlic cloves, minced
- 1 red onion, chopped
- A few thyme springs

Directions:

⇒ In a baking dish, mix potatoes with tomatoes, onion, bell pepper, garlic, a pinch of sea salt and pepper and stir gently.

⇒ Heat up a pan over high heat, add turkey mince, brown it for 15 minutes side and transfer on top of veggies in the baking dish.

⇒ Add thyme, introduce in the oven at 400 degrees F and bake for 45 minutes.

⇒ Divide between plates and serve hot.

Nutrition: calories 306, fat 10,8, carbs 28,4, fiber 4,8, protein 28,2

62) Steak and Veggies

Preparation Time: 10 minutes   **Cooking Time: 20 minutes**   **Servings:4**

Ingredients:

- 3 sweet potatoes, cubed
- 1 yellow onion, chopped
- 12 mini bell peppers, chopped
- 4 medium round steaks
- ½ cup sun dried tomatoes, chopped
- 1 tablespoon sweet paprika
- 2 tablespoons balsamic vinegar
- Juice of 1 lemon

- 1 tablespoons oregano, dried
- ¼ cup olive oil+ a drizzle
- 1 lemon, sliced
- ¼ cup kalamata olives, pitted and chopped
- 4 dill springs
- 2 garlic cloves, minced
- A pinch of sea salt and black pepper

Directions:

⇒ Heat up a pan with a drizzle of oil over medium-high heat, add steaks, season them with salt and some black pepper, brown them for 2 minutes on each side and transfer to a baking dish.

⇒ Heat up the pan again over medium-high heat, add sweet potatoes, cook them for 4 minutes and add them to the baking dish.

⇒ Also add bell peppers, tomatoes, onion, olives and lemon slices.

⇒ Meanwhile, in a bowl, mix lemon juice with rest of the olive oil, vinegar, garlic, paprika and oregano and whisk well.

⇒ Pour this over steak and veggies, add dill springs on top, toss to coat, place in the oven at 425 degrees F and bake for 12 minutes.

⇒ Divide steak and veggies between plates and serve.

Nutrition: calories 869, fat 30,8, fiber 10,9, carbs 56,5, protein 89,1

63) Steaks and Pico de Gallo

Preparation Time: 10 minutes   **Cooking Time: 15 minutes**   **Servings:4**

Ingredients:

- 2 tablespoons chili powder
- 4 medium sirloin steaks
- 1 teaspoon cumin, ground
- ½ tablespoon sweet paprika
- 1 teaspoon onion powder
- 1 teaspoon garlic powder
- A pinch of sea salt and black pepper

For the Pico de gallo:

- 1 small red onion, chopped

- 2 tomatoes, chopped
- 2 garlic cloves, minced
- 2 tablespoons lime juice
- 1 small green bell pepper, chopped
- 1 jalapeno, chopped
- ¼ cup cilantro, chopped
- ¼ teaspoon cumin, ground
- Black pepper to taste

Directions:

⇒ In a bowl, mix chili powder with a pinch of salt, black pepper, onion powder, garlic powder, paprika and 1 teaspoon cumin and stir well.

⇒ Season steaks with this mix, rub well and place them on preheated grill over medium high heat.

⇒ Cook steaks for 5 minutes on each side and divide them between plates.

⇒ In a bowl, mix red onion with tomatoes, garlic, lime juice, bell pepper, jalapeno, cilantro, black pepper to taste and ¼ teaspoon cumin and stir well.

⇒ Top steaks with this mix and serve.

Nutrition: calories 285, fat 9, fiber 3,1 carbs 10,2, protein 40,5

64) Coffee Steaks

Preparation Time: 10 minutes   **Cooking Time: 10 minutes**   **Servings:4**

Ingredients:

- 1 and ½ tablespoons coffee, ground
- 4 rib eye steaks
- ½ tablespoon sweet paprika
- 2 tablespoons chili powder
- 2 teaspoons garlic powder

- 2 teaspoons onion powder
- ¼ teaspoon ginger, ground
- ¼ teaspoon, coriander, ground
- A pinch of cayenne pepper
- Black pepper to the taste

Directions:

⇒ In a bowl, mix coffee with paprika, chili powder, garlic powder, onion powder, ginger, coriander, cayenne and black pepper and stir well.

⇒ Rub steaks with the coffee mix, place them on your preheated grill over medium high heat, cook them for 5 minutes on each side and divide between plates.

⇒ Leave steaks to cool down for 5 minutes before serving them with a side salad!

Nutrition: calories 621, fat 50, fiber 0, carbs 0, protein 40

65) Beef Casserolle

Preparation Time: 10 minutes   Cooking Time: 6 hours   **Servings: 6**

Ingredients:

- 1 red bell pepper, chopped
- 1 eggplant, sliced lengthwise
- 2 zucchinis, sliced lengthwise
- 1 pound beef, ground
- 2 cups tomatoes, chopped
- 2 teaspoons oregano, dried
- 4 cups tomato sauce
- ¼ cup basil, chopped

- 2 garlic cloves, minced
- 1 yellow onion, chopped
- 2 tablespoons tomato paste
- 1 tablespoon parsley, chopped
- 2 tablespoons olive oil
- A pinch of sea salt
- Black pepper to taste

Directions:

⇒ Heat up a pan with the oil over medium-high heat, add onion and garlic, stir and cook for 2 minutes.

⇒ Add beef, stir and brown for 5 minutes more.

⇒ Add bell pepper, tomatoes, oregano, basil, tomato paste and parsley, stir and cook for 4 minutes more.

⇒ Add tomato sauce, black pepper to taste and a pinch of salt and stir well again.

⇒ Arrange layers of eggplant and zucchini slices with the sauce you've made in your slow cooker.

⇒ Cover and cook on Low for 4 hours and 45 minutes.

⇒ Divide your lasagna between plates and serve.

Nutrition: calories 281, fat 10,2, fiber 7,7, carbs 22,7, protein 28

Chapter 7 -   Seafood & Fish Recipes

66) Sesame Tuna

Preparation Time: 15 minutes   **Cooking Time: 10 minutes**   **Servings:4**

Ingredients:

- 1 teaspoon fennel seeds
- 1 teaspoon mustard seeds
- 4 medium tuna steaks
- ¼ teaspoon black peppercorns
- A pinch of sea salt
- Black pepper to taste
- 4 tablespoons sesame seeds, toasted
- 3 tablespoons coconut oil, melted

Directions:

⇒ In your grinder, mix peppercorns with fennel, mustard seeds, sesame seeds, a pinch of sea salt, pepper to taste and grind well.

⇒ Spread this mix on a plate, add tuna steaks and toss to coat.

⇒ Heat up a pan with the oil over medium-high heat, add tuna steaks and cook for 3 minutes on each side.

⇒ Divide between plates and serve with a side salad.

Nutrition: calories 458, fat 25,7, carbs 2,7, fiber 1,4, protein 52,8

67) Lime Tartar

Preparation Time: 15 minutes   **Cooking Time: 0 minutes**   **Servings:4**

Ingredients:

- 7 ounces smoked salmon, minced
- 14 ounces salmon fillet, cut into very small cubes
- 3 tablespoons red onion, minced
- 2 tablespoons pickled cucumber, minced
- Zest and juice from 1 lemon
- 1 garlic clove, finely minced
- 2 tablespoons basil, minced
- 2 teaspoons oregano, dried
- Black pepper to taste
- 2 tablespoons mint leaves, minced
- 2 tablespoons Dijon mustard
- 5 tablespoons extra virgin olive oil
- Lime wedges for serving

Directions:

⇒ In a bowl, combine all the ingredients, stir well and keep in the fridge for 15 minutes

⇒ Divide the tartar between plates and serve with lime wedges on the side.

Nutrition: calories 361, fat 26,3, carbs 5,1, fiber 1,5, protein 29,2

68) Salmon and Onion Mix

Preparation Time: 10 minutes   **Cooking Time: 15 minutes**   **Servings:4**

Ingredients:

- 2 red onions, cut into wedges
- 3 peaches, cut into wedges
- 4 salmon steaks
- 1 teaspoon thyme, chopped
- 1 tablespoon ginger, grated
- A pinch of sea salt
- Black pepper to taste
- 1 tablespoon balsamic vinegar
- 3 tablespoons extra virgin olive oil

Directions:

⇒ In a bowl, mix the ginger, vinegar, thyme, a pinch of sea salt, pepper and olive oil and whisk very well.

⇒ In another bowl, mix peaches with onion, salt and pepper and toss to coat.

⇒ Heat up your kitchen grill over medium-high heat, add salmon steaks, season with salt and pepper, grill for 6 minutes on each side and divide between plates.

⇒ Add peaches and onions to grill, cook for 4 minutes on each side and transfer next to salmon on plates.

⇒ Drizzle the vinaigrette you've made all over the salmon and peaches mix and serve.

Nutrition: calories 398, fat 22, carbs 16,8, fiber 3,2, protein 36,3

69) Shrimp and Radish Cakes

Preparation Time: 15 minutes   **Cooking Time: 15 minutes**   **Servings:4**

Ingredients:

- 2 tablespoons cilantro, chopped
- 1 and ½ pounds shrimp, peeled and deveined
- 2 tablespoons chives, chopped
- Black pepper to taste
- 1 garlic clove, minced
- ¼ cup radishes, minced
- 1 teaspoon lemon zest, grated
- ¼ cup celery, minced
- 1 egg, whisked
- 1 tablespoon lemon juice
- ¼ cup almond meal

For the salsa:

- 1 avocado, pitted, peeled and chopped
- 1 cup pineapple, chopped
- 2 tablespoons red onion, chopped
- ¼ cup bell peppers, chopped
- 1 tablespoon lime juice
- 1 tablespoon cilantro, finely chopped
- A pinch of sea salt
- Black pepper to taste

Directions:

⇒ In a bowl, mix the pineapple with avocado, bell peppers, 2 tablespoons red onion, 1 tablespoon lime juice, pepper to taste and 1 tablespoon cilantro, stir well and keep in the fridge for now.

⇒ In your food processor, mix shrimp with 2 tablespoons cilantro, chives, and garlic and blend well.

⇒ Transfer to a bowl and mix with radishes, celery, lemon zest, lemon juice, egg, almond meal, a pinch of sea salt and pepper to taste and stir well.

⇒ Shape 4 burgers, place them on preheated grill over medium-high heat and cook for 5 minutes on each side.

⇒ Divide shrimp burgers between plates and serve with the salsa you've made earlier on the side.

Nutrition: calories 406, fat 17,2, carbs 16,1, fiber 5,3, protein 46,8

70) Basil Scallops Mix

Preparation Time: 15 minutes   **Cooking Time: 0 minutes**   **Servings:2**

Ingredients:

- 6 scallops, diced
- A pinch of sea salt
- Black pepper to taste
- 3 strawberries, chopped

- 1 tablespoon extra-virgin olive oil
- 1 tablespoon green onions, minced
- Juice from ½ lemon
- ½ tablespoon basil leaves, finely chopped

Directions:

⇒ In a bowl, mix all the ingredients, toss and keep in the fridge for 15 minutes.

⇒ Keep the tartar in the fridge until ready to serve.

Nutrition: calories 149, fat 7,8, carbs 4,8, fiber 0,5, protein 15,3

71) Creole Shrimp Mix

Preparation Time: 10 minutes   **Cooking Time: 10 minutes**   Servings:4

Ingredients:

- ½ pound turkey meat, already cooked and sliced
- ½ pound shrimp, peeled and deveined
- 2 tablespoons extra virgin olive oil
- 2 zucchinis, cubed
- A pinch of sea salt
- Black pepper to taste

For the Creole seasoning:

- ½ tablespoon garlic powder
- 2 tablespoons paprika
- ½ tablespoon onion powder
- ¼ tablespoon oregano, dried
- ½ tablespoon chili powder
- ¼ tablespoon thyme, dried

Directions:

⇒ In a bowl, mix paprika with garlic powder, onion one, chili powder, oregano, and thyme and stir well.

⇒ In another bowl, mix shrimp with turkey meat, zucchini, and oil and toss to coat.

⇒ Pour paprika mix over shrimp mix and stir well.

⇒ Arrange turkey, shrimp, and zucchini on skewers alternating pieces, season with a pinch of sea salt and black pepper, place them on preheated grill over medium-high heat and cook for 8 minutes, flipping skewers from time to time.

⇒ Divide the skewers between plates and serve.

Nutrition: calories 260, fat 11,7, fiber 3, carbs 8,3, protein 31,7

72) Orange Salmon Bites

Preparation Time: 10 minutes   **Cooking Time: 15 minutes**   Servings:4

Ingredients:

- 1 pound wild salmon, skinless, boneless and cubed
- 2 Meyer lemons, sliced
- ¼ cup balsamic vinegar

- ¼ cup orange juice
- A pinch of pink salt
- Black pepper to taste

Directions:

⇒ Heat up a small saucepan with the vinegar over medium heat, add the orange juice, stir, bring to a simmer for 1 minute and take off the heat.

⇒ Skewer salmon cubes and lemon slices, season with salt and black pepper, brush them with half of the vinegar mix, place on preheated grill over medium heat, cook for 4 minutes on each side.

⇒ Brush skewers with the rest of the vinegar mix, grill for 1 minute more, divide between plates and serve.

Nutrition: calories 290, fat 12,6, fiber 3, carbs 11,8, protein 40,3

73) Sushi Tuna Mix

Preparation Time: 10 minutes   **Cooking Time: 5 minutes**   **Servings: 4**

Ingredients:

- 1 small red onion, chopped
- ½ cup cilantro, chopped
- 1/3 cup olive oil+ 2 tablespoons
- 1 jalapeno pepper, chopped
- 2 tablespoons basil, chopped
- 3 tablespoons vinegar
- 3 garlic cloves, minced
- 1 teaspoon red pepper flakes
- 1 teaspoon thyme, chopped
- A pinch of sea salt
- Black pepper to taste
- 1 pound sushi grade tuna
- 2 avocados, pitted, peeled and chopped
- 6 ounces arugula

Directions:

⇒ In a bowl, mix 1/3 cup oil with onion, jalapeno, cilantro, basil, vinegar, garlic, parsley, pepper flakes, thyme, a pinch of salt and black pepper and whisk well.

⇒ Heat up a pan with the rest of the oil over medium-high heat, add tuna, season salt and black pepper, cook for 2 minutes on each side, transfer to a cutting board, leave aside to cool down and slice.

⇒ In a bowl, mix arugula with half of the chimichurri sauce you've made earlier, toss to coat well and divide between plates.

⇒ Also divide tuna slices, and avocado pieces and drizzle the rest of the sauce on top.

Nutrition: calories 938, fat 62,8, fiber 10, carbs 51,9, protein 43,8

74) Chili Salmon

Preparation Time: 10 minutes   **Cooking Time: 15 minutes**   **Servings: 12**

Ingredients:

- 1 and ¼ cups coconut, shredded
- 1 pound salmon meat, cubed
- 1/3 cup coconut flour
- A pinch of sea salt
- Black pepper to taste
- 1 egg
- 2 tablespoons coconut oil
- ¼ cup water
- 4 red chilies, chopped
- 3 garlic cloves, minced
- ¼ cup balsamic vinegar
- ½ cup honey

Directions:

⇒ In another bowl, whisk the egg with black pepper.

⇒ Put coconut in a third bowl.

⇒ Dip salmon cubes in flour, egg and coconut and place them all on a working surface.

⇒ Heat up a pan with the oil over medium-high heat, add salmon cubes, fry them for 3 minutes on each side, transfer them to paper towels, drain grease and divide them between plates.

⇒ Heat up a pan with the water over medium-high heat.

⇒ Add chilies, cloves, vinegar, honey and agar agar, stir well, bring to a gentle boil and simmer until all ingredients combine.

⇒ Drizzle this over salmon cubes and serve.

Nutrition: calories 180, fat 8,5, fiber 0,9, carbs 19,7, protein 7,7

75) Clams and Apple Mix

Preparation Time: 10 minutes   **Cooking Time: 12 minutes**   **Servings:2**

Ingredients:

- 3 tablespoons ghee, melted
- 2 pound little clams, scrubbed
- 1 shallot, minced
- 2 garlic cloves, minced

- 1 cup cider
- 1 apple, cored and chopped
- Juice of ½ lemon

Directions:

⇒ Heat up a pan with the ghee over medium-high heat, add the shallot and garlic, stir and cook for 3 minutes.

⇒ Add cider, stir well and cook for 1 minute.

⇒ Add clams and thyme, cover and simmer for 5 minutes.

⇒ Add apple and lemon juice, stir, divide everything into bowls and serve.

Nutrition: calories 610, fat 23,6, fiber 2,9, carbs 43,7, protein 55,1

76) Fennel Salmon Mix

Preparation Time: 10 minutes   **Cooking Time: 30 minutes**   **Servings:6**

Ingredients:

- 2 tablespoons ghee, melted
- A pinch of sea salt
- Black pepper to taste
- 3 cups chicken stock

- ½ teaspoon fennel seeds
- 1 teaspoon mustard seeds
- 2 apples, cored, peeled and cubed
- 4 salmon fillets, skin on and bone in

Directions:

⇒ Put the stock in a pot, heat up over medium heat, add mustard seeds, a pinch of salt, black pepper and fennel seeds, stir and boil for 25 minutes.

⇒ Strain this into a bowl, add half of the ghee, stir well and leave aside for now.

⇒ Heat up a pan with the rest of the ghee over medium heat, add apple pieces, stir and cook for 6 minutes.

⇒ Brush salmon pieces with some of the stock mix, season with a pinch of salt and black pepper, place on a lined baking sheet, also add apple pieces, introduce everything in the oven at 350 degrees F and bake for 25 minutes.

⇒ Divide salmon between plates and serve with the rest of the stock drizzled on top.

Nutrition: calories 241, fat 12,2, fiber 2, carbs 10,9, protein 23,7

77) Shrimp and Parsley Mix

Preparation Time: 10 minutes   **Cooking Time: 5 minutes**   **Servings:4**

Ingredients:

- 1 pound big shrimp, peeled and deveined
- 2 teaspoons olive oil
- 1 cup cilantro, chopped
- 1 cup parsley, chopped
- Juice from 2 limes

- ½ cup olive oil
- ¼ cup yellow onion, chopped
- A pinch of sea salt
- ½ teaspoon smoked paprika
- 2 garlic cloves, minced

Directions:

⇒ Heat up a pan with 2 teaspoons olive oil over medium heat, add shrimp, cook them for 5 minutes and reduce heat to low.

⇒ In a food processor, mix ½ cup oil with onion, sea salt, paprika, garlic, lime juice, parsley and cilantro and pulse well.

⇒ Divide shrimp on plates, top with the chimichurri and serve.

Nutrition: calories 374, fat 26,9, fiber 1, carbs 4,3, protein 30,5

78) Scallops Salad

Preparation Time: 10 minutes   **Cooking Time: 13 minutes**   **Servings:4**

Ingredients:

- 1 shallot, minced
- 3 garlic cloves, minced
- 1 and ½ cups chicken stock
- ¼ cup walnuts, toasted and chopped
- 1 and ½ cups grapes, halved

- 2 cups spinach
- 1 tablespoon avocado oil
- 1 pound scallops
- A pinch of sea salt
- Black pepper to taste

Directions:

⇒ Heat up a pan with the oil over medium heat, add the shallot and the garlic, stir and cook for 2 minutes.

⇒ Add the walnuts, grapes, salt and pepper, stir and cook for 3 more minutes.

⇒ Add the scallops and cook them for 2 minutes on each side.

⇒ Add the spinach, toss, cook everything for 3 more minutes, divide everything into bowls and serve.

Nutrition: calories 205, fat 7,4, fiber 1,5, carbs 17,5, protein 24,9

79) Crab and Sauce

Preparation Time: 10 minutes   **Cooking Time: 7 minutes**   **Servings:8**

Ingredients:

- 1 cup crab meat
- 2 tablespoons parsley, chopped
- 2 tablespoons old bay seasoning
- 2 teaspoons Dijon mustard
- 1 egg, whisked
- 1 tablespoons lemon juice
- 2 tablespoons coconut oil

- 1 and ½ tablespoons coconut flour

  For the sauce:
- 1 tablespoon olive oil
- ¼ cup roasted red peppers
- 1 tablespoon lemon juice
- ¼ cup avocado, peeled and chopped

Directions:

⇒ In a bowl, mix crabmeat with old bay seasoning, parsley, mustard, egg, 1 tablespoon lemon juice and coconut flour and stir everything very well.

⇒ Shape 8 patties from this mix and place them on a plate.

⇒ Heat up a pan with 2 tablespoons coconut oil over medium-high heat, add crab patties, cook for 3 minutes on each side and divide between plates.

⇒ In a food processor, mix olive oil with red peppers, avocado and 1 tablespoon lemon juice and blend well.

⇒ Spread this on the crab patties and serve.

Nutrition: calories 69, fat 6,8, fiber 0,5, carbs 1,1, protein 1,4

Chapter 8 -   Salad Recipes

80) Broccoli and Beef Salad

Preparation Time: 10 minutes   **Cooking Time: 10 minutes**   **Servings:4**

Ingredients:

- 1 pound organic beef steak, cut into strips
- 3 cups broccoli, florets separated
- 8 cups baby salad greens
- 1 red onion, sliced
- 1 red bell pepper, sliced
- For the vinaigrette:
- 1 tablespoon ginger, minced

- A pinch of sea salt
- Black pepper to taste
- ½ cup extra virgin olive oil
- 2 tablespoons lime juice
- 1 tablespoon balsamic vinegar
- 2 tablespoons shallots, finely chopped

Directions:

⇒ In a bowl, mix ginger with oil, lime juice, vinegar, shallots, a pinch of sea salt and pepper to taste and stir well.

⇒ Heat up a pan over medium-high heat, add 2 tablespoons of vinaigrette, warm up, add broccoli and cook for 3 minutes.

⇒ Add beef, stir and cook for 4 more minutes and take off heat.

⇒ In a salad bowl, mix salad greens with onion, bell pepper, broccoli, and beef.

⇒ Add some black pepper, drizzle the rest of the vinaigrette, toss to coat and serve.

Nutrition: calories 513, fat 32,7, carbs 17,6, fiber 5, protein 39,2

81) Dijon Spinach Salad

Preparation Time: 10 minutes   **Cooking Time: 20 minutes**   **Servings:4**

Ingredients:

- 2 red onions, cut into medium wedges
- 1 butternut squash, cut into medium wedges
- 6 cups spinach
- 4 parsnips, cut into medium wedges
- Black pepper to taste
- 2 tablespoons balsamic vinegar

- 1/3 cup nuts, roasted
- 1 teaspoon Dijon mustard
- ½ tablespoons oregano, dried
- 1 garlic clove, minced
- 6 tablespoons extra virgin olive oil

Directions:

⇒ Put the squash, onions, and parsnips in a baking dish.

⇒ Drizzle half of the oil, sprinkle oregano and pepper to the taste, toss to coat, place in the oven at 400 degrees F and bake for 10 minutes.

⇒ Take veggies out of the oven, turn them and bake for another 10 minutes.

⇒ In a bowl, mix vinegar with the rest of the oil, garlic, mustard and pepper to taste and stir very well.

⇒ Put spinach in a salad bowl, add roasted veggies, pour salad dressing, sprinkle nuts, toss to coat and serve warm.

Nutrition: calories 401, fat 27,7, carbs 38,4, fiber 10,7, protein 6

82) Chicken and Arugula Salad

Preparation Time: 10 minutes   **Cooking Time: 35 minutes**   **Servings:4**

Ingredients:

- 2 tablespoons ghee, melted
- 1 tablespoon balsamic vinegar
- 1 zucchini, cubed
- 2 small shallots, peeled, chopped
- 4 eggs
- 2 lettuce heads, leaves, torn
- 2 cups chicken meat, already cooked and shredded
- 4 cups arugula
- 1 small red onion, finely chopped
- 1/3 cup cranberries
- A pinch of sea salt

- Black pepper to taste
- A pinch of garlic powder
- 1/3 cup pecans, chopped
- 2 apples, chopped
- 2 tablespoons maple syrup
- 1 tablespoon apple cider vinegar
- 1 teaspoon shallot, minced
- 1 teaspoon mustard
- 1 teaspoon garlic, minced
- ¼ cup extra virgin olive oil

Directions:

⇒ Spread zucchini cubes on a lined baking sheet, sprinkle with a pinch of sea salt, pepper, garlic powder, drizzle balsamic vinegar and add ghee, toss to coat, place in the oven at 400 degrees F and bake for 25 minutes.

⇒ Meanwhile, put eggs in a saucepan, add water to cover, bring to a boil over medium-high heat, boil for 15 minutes, drain, place in a bowl filled with ice water, leave aside to cool down, peel them, chop and put in a salad bowl. Heat up a pan over medium-high heat, add shallots, brown for 7 minutes, take off heat, leave to cool down and add to the same bowl with the eggs.

⇒ Add lettuce leaves, arugula, chicken, onion, pecans, apple pieces, roasted squash cubes, and cranberries. In a small bowl, mix maple syrup with apple cider vinegar, mustard, garlic, shallot, olive oil and pepper and whisk very well.

⇒ Pour this over salad, toss to coat and serve.

Nutrition: calories 628, fat 42, carbs 36,9, fiber 7,3, protein 30,5

83) Cayenne Scallops and Avocado Salad

Preparation Time: 10 minutes   **Cooking Time: 7 minutes**   **Servings:4**

Ingredients:

- 1 pound bay scallops
- 2 teaspoons cayenne pepper
- Black pepper to taste
- 3 tablespoons lemon juice
- 1 tablespoon homemade mayonnaise
- 1 teaspoon mustard
- A pinch of cayenne pepper

- ½ cup extra virgin olive oil
- 1 garlic clove, minced
- 2 handfuls mixed greens
- 1 avocado, pitted, peeled and cubed
- 1 red bell pepper, cut into thin strips
- 3 tablespoons melted coconut oil

Directions:

⇒ In a salad bowl, mix salad greens with avocado and pepper and leave aside for now.

⇒ In a bowl, mix lemon juice with mustard, garlic, mayo, pepper and a pinch of cayenne, stir well and leave aside.

⇒ Add olive oil gradually and whisk well again.

⇒ Rinse and pat dry scallops, put them in another bowl, add pepper to taste and 2 teaspoons cayenne and toss to coat.

⇒ Heat up a pan with the coconut oil over medium-high heat, add scallops, cook for 2 minutes on each side and transfer them to the bowl with the veggies.

⇒ Add mustard dressing you've made, toss to coat and serve.

Nutrition: calories 592, fat 46,3, carbs 23,8, fiber 28,9, protein 24,3

84) Pork and Lettuce Salad

Preparation Time: 10 minutes   **Cooking Time: 5 minutes**   **Servings:4**

Ingredients:

- 2 lettuce heads, torn
- 2 cups pork, already cooked and shredded
- 1 avocado, pitted, peeled and chopped
- 1 cup cherry tomatoes, cut in halves
- 1 green bell pepper, sliced
- 2 green onions, thinly sliced
- A pinch of sea salt

- Black pepper to taste
- Juice of ½ lime
- 1 tablespoon apple cider vinegar
- ¼ cup BBQ sauce
- 2 tablespoons extra virgin olive oil

Directions:

⇒ In a small bowl, mix oil with lime juice, vinegar, black pepper and BBQ sauce and whisk well.

⇒ Heat up a pan over medium heat, add pork meat and heat it up.

⇒ Meanwhile, in a salad bowl, mix lettuce leaves with tomatoes, bell pepper, avocado and green onions.

⇒ Add pork, drizzle the BBQ dressing, toss to coat and serve.

Nutrition: calories 349, fat 20,2, carbs 19,9, fiber 5,7, protein 24,3

85) Shrimp and Crab Salad

Preparation Time: 3 hours   **Cooking Time: 0 minutes**   **Servings:6**

Ingredients:

- 8 ounces, baby shrimp, already cooked, peeled, deveined and chopped
- 8 ounces crab meat, already cooked
- 2/3 cup homemade mayonnaise
- 2/3 cup yellow onion, chopped
- 2/3 cup celery, chopped

- 2 tablespoons Dijon mustard
- Black pepper to taste
- ¼ teaspoon onion powder
- ½ teaspoon garlic powder
- 1 tablespoon hot sauce

Directions:

⇒ In a salad bowl, mix shrimp with crab meat, onion, and celery.

⇒ In another bowl, mix mayo with mustard, pepper, onion powder, garlic powder and hot sauce and stir well.

⇒ Pour this over seafood salad, toss to coat and keep in the fridge for 3 hours before you serve it.

Nutrition: calories 198, fat 9,9, carbs 9, fiber 0,6, protein 16,8

86) Cilantro Beef Salad

Preparation Time: 10 minutes   **Cooking Time: 15 minutes**   **Servings:4**

Ingredients:

- 1 tablespoon chili powder
- 1 teaspoon onion powder
- ½ teaspoon garlic powder
- 1 teaspoon cumin, ground
- 2 teaspoons paprika
- 3 tablespoons olive oil
- A pinch of cayenne pepper
- 1 pound beef, ground
- 3 cups cilantro, chopped

- Juice from 1 lime
- A pinch of sea salt
- Black pepper to taste
- 1 romaine lettuce head, chopped
- 1 avocado, pitted, peeled and chopped
- 1 small red onion, chopped
- Some black olives, pitted and chopped
- 1 red bell pepper, chopped
- ½ cup Pico de gallo

Directions:

⇒ In a bowl, mix chili powder with paprika, onion and garlic powder, ½ teaspoon cumin, cayenne and some black pepper and stir.

⇒ Heat up a pan with 1 tablespoon oil over medium heat, add beef, stir and cook for 7 minutes.

⇒ Add spice mix, stir and cook until meat is done.

⇒ Meanwhile, in your food processor, blend 1 cup cilantro with lime juice, ½ teaspoon cumin, a pinch of salt, black pepper to taste and 2 tablespoons oil and pulse well.

⇒ In a salad bowl, mix lettuce leaves with avocado, 2 cups cilantro, onion, bell pepper, olives and Pico de gallo and stir.

⇒ Divide this between plates, top with beef and drizzle the salad dressing on top.

Nutrition: calories 464, fat 29,4, fiber 6,2, carbs 15,8, protein 27,1

87) Lemon Berries and Honeydew Salad

Preparation Time: 10 minutes   **Cooking Time: 0 minutes**   **Servings:6**

Ingredients:

- 1 cup blackberries, halved
- 2 cups honeydew, sliced
- 8 ounces prosciutto
- 3 tablespoons chives, chopped
- Juice of 1 lemon

- Zest from 1 lemon
- 1 shallot, chopped
- 2 cup cantaloupe, sliced
- A pinch of sea salt
- Black pepper to taste

Directions:

⇒ In a large salad bowl, mix blackberries with prosciutto, honeydew, cantaloupe, chives, lemon juice and zest, shallot, a pinch of sea salt and black pepper to taste, toss to coat and serve cold.

Nutrition: calories 107, fat 2,4, fiber 2,3, carbs 13,3, protein 9,1

88) Brussels Sprouts and Pecan Salad

Preparation Time: 10 minutes   **Cooking Time: 7 minutes**   **Servings:2**

Ingredients:

- 1 red onion, chopped
- 12 Brussels sprouts, sliced
- A pinch of sea salt
- Black pepper to taste
- 1 tablespoon olive oil

- 1/3 cup pecans, chopped
- ¼ cup raisins
- 2/3 cup hemp seeds
- ½ red apple, cored and chopped

Directions:

⇒ Heat up a pan with the oil over medium heat, add onion, stir and cook for a few minutes.

⇒ Add Brussels sprouts, cook for 4 minutes, take off heat and leave aside to cool down.

⇒ Add apple pieces, hemp seeds, raisins, a pinch of sea salt, black pepper and pecans, stir salad and serve.

Nutrition: calories 522, fat 34,8, fiber 10,2, carbs 42,1, protein 19,2

89) Lime Kale and Lettuce Salad

Preparation Time: 10 minutes   **Cooking Time: 0 minutes**   **Servings:1**

Ingredients:

- 1 carrot, grated
- A handful kale, chopped
- 1 small lettuce head, chopped
- 1 tablespoon tahini paste
- 1 tablespoon olive oil

- A pinch of sea salt
- Black pepper to taste
- Juice of ½ lime
- A pinch of garlic powder

Directions:

⇒ In a salad bowl, mix carrots with kale and lettuce leaves.

⇒ In a blender, mix tahini with a pinch of salt, black pepper, garlic powder, lime juice and oil and pulse well.

⇒ Pour this over salad, toss to coat well and serve.

Nutrition: calories 264, fat 22,2, fiber 3,8, carbs 16,9, protein 4,2

90) Chicken and Eggs Salad

Preparation Time: 10 minutes   **Cooking Time: 0 minutes**   **Servings:2**

Ingredients:

- 1 smoked chicken breast, sliced
- 2 handfuls lettuce leaves, torn
- 1 avocado, pitted, peeled and cubed

- 2 eggs, hard-boiled and halved
- A handful walnuts, chopped
- 2 tablespoons flaxseed oil

Directions:

⇒ In a salad bowl, mix lettuce with avocado, walnuts and chicken slices and toss.

⇒ Add eggs and oil, toss gently and serve.

Nutrition: calories 678, fat 49,7, fiber 10,7, carbs 20,9, protein 34,7

91) Balsamic Potato and Turkey Salad

Preparation Time: 10 minutes   **Cooking Time: 30 minutes**   **Servings:4**

Ingredients:

- 3 sweet potatoes, cubed
- 2 tablespoons coconut oil
- 4 garlic cloves, minced
- ½ pound turkey fillet, cut into thin slices
- Juice from 1 lime
- A pinch of sea salt
- Black pepper to taste

- 2 tablespoons balsamic vinegar
- 2 tablespoons olive oil
- A handful dill, chopped
- 2 green onions, chopped
- A pinch of cinnamon, ground
- A pinch of red pepper flakes

Directions:

⇒ Arrange turkey and sweet potatoes on a lined baking sheet, add garlic and coconut oil, toss well, place in the oven at 375 degrees F and bake for 30 minutes.

⇒ Meanwhile, in a bowl, mix vinegar with lime juice, olive oil, green onions, pepper flakes, dill, a pinch of sea salt, black pepper and cinnamon and stir well.

⇒ Transfer turkey and sweet potatoes to a salad bowl, add salad dressing, toss well and serve.

Nutrition: calories 316, fat 4,4, fiber 5,1, carbs 34,5, protein 13,4

92) Chicken and Olives Salad

Preparation Time: 10 minutes   **Cooking Time: 0 minutes**   **Servings:1**

Ingredients:

- 1 chicken breast, cooked and sliced
- 1 medium lettuce head, chopped
- 1 sweet potato, boiled and cubed
- 1 tablespoon pumpkin seeds

- 6 black olives, pitted and chopped
- 1 tablespoon olive oil
- 1 tablespoon balsamic vinegar

Directions:

⇒ In a salad bowl, mix chicken breast slices with lettuce, sweet potato, pumpkin seeds, olives, olive oil and balsamic vinegar, stir well and serve right away.

⇒

Nutrition: calories 760, fat 30,4, fiber 8,4, carbs 43,1, protein 78,3

93) Salmon and Cucumber Salad

Preparation Time: 10 minutes   **Cooking Time: 5 minutes**   **Servings:2**

Ingredients:

- 1 lettuce head, chopped
- 2 salmon fillets
- 1 tablespoon olive oil
- 1 tablespoon coconut aminos

- 1 avocado, pitted, peeled and sliced
- 1 cucumber, sliced
- A pinch of sea salt
- Black pepper to taste

Directions:

⇒ Heat up a pan with the oil over medium-high heat, add salmon fillets skin side down, cook for 3 minutes, flip and cook for 2 minutes more.

⇒ In a salad bowl, mix lettuce with cucumber, avocado, a pinch of salt, black pepper and coconut aminos and stir.

⇒ Flake salmon using a fork, add to salad, drizzle some of the oil from the pan, toss to coat and serve.

Nutrition: calories 550, fat 38,1, fiber 8,5, carbs 20, protein 38,2

94) Lettuce, Kale and Radish Salad

Preparation Time: 10 minutes   **Cooking Time: 0 minutes**   **Servings:3**

Ingredients:

- 1 lettuce head, chopped
- A handful kale, chopped
- A handful steamed broccoli
- A handful walnuts, chopped
- 8 cherry tomatoes, halved
- A handful radishes, chopped
- 1 tablespoon lemon juice
- 8 dates, chopped
- A drizzle of olive oil

Directions:

⇒ In a salad bowl, mix lettuce with kale, broccoli, walnuts, tomatoes, radishes and dates.

⇒ In smaller bowl, mix lemon juice with olive oil and whisk well.

⇒ Add this to salad, toss to coat and serve.

Nutrition: calories 771, fat 35,2, fiber 36,2, carbs 112,4, protein 21,4

95) Tomato and Mayo Salad

Preparation Time: 10 minutes   **Cooking Time: 0 minutes**   **Servings:4**

Ingredients:

- 1 bunch kale, chopped
- 12 cherry tomatoes, halved
- 2 handfuls microgreens
- 3 tablespoons Paleo mayonnaise
- 1 teaspoon mustard

Directions:

⇒ In a salad bowl, mix tomatoes with greens and kale.

⇒ In a small bowl, mix mayo with mustard and whisk well.

⇒ Add this to salad, toss to coat and serve.

Nutrition: calories 145, fat 8,5, fiber 4,9, carbs 16, protein 4

Chapter 9 - 　　Dessert Recipes

96) Maple Rhubarb Bowls

Preparation Time: 10 minutes   **Cooking Time: 5 minutes**   **Servings:3**

Ingredients:

- Juice of 1 lemon
- Some thin lemon zest strips
- 1 and ½ cup maple syrup
- 4 and ½ cups rhubarbs cut into medium pieces.
- 1 vanilla bean
- 1 and ½ cups water

Directions:

⇒ Put the water in a saucepan.

⇒ Add maple syrup, vanilla bean, lemon juice and lemon zest.

⇒ Stir, bring to a boil and add rhubarb.

⇒ Reduce heat, simmer for 5 minutes, take off heat and transfer rhubarb to a bowl.

⇒ Allow liquid to cool down, discard vanilla bean and serve.

Nutrition: calories 297, fat 0,6, fiber 2,8, carbs 75,3, protein 1,4

97) Maple Cobbler

Preparation Time: 10 minutes   **Cooking Time: 30 minutes**   **Servings:5**

Ingredients:

- ¾ cup maple syrup
- 6 cups strawberries, halved
- 1 tablespoon lemon juice
- ½ cup coconut flour
- 1/4 teaspoon baking soda
- ½ cup water
- 3 and ½ tablespoons coconut oil
- A drizzle of avocado oil

Directions:

⇒ Grease a baking dish with a drizzle of avocado oil and leave aside.

⇒ In a bowl, mix strawberries with maple syrup, sprinkle some flour and add lemon juice.

⇒ Stir very well and pour into baking dish.

⇒ In another bowl, mix flour with baking soda and stir well.

⇒ Add coconut and mix until the whole thing crumbles in your hands.

⇒ Add ½ cup water and spread over strawberries.

⇒ Place in the oven at 375 degrees F and bake for 30 minutes.

⇒ Take cobbler out of the oven, leave aside for 10 minutes and then serve.

Nutrition: calories 318, fat 11,2, fiber 9,5, carbs 55, protein 3,2

98) Cocoa Almond Bowls

Preparation Time: 3 hours   **Cooking Time:**   **Servings:4**

Ingredients:

- 1 cup almond milk
- 2 avocados, peeled and pitted
- ¾ cup cocoa powder
- 1 teaspoon vanilla extract
- ¾ cup maple syrup
- ¼ teaspoon cinnamon
- Walnuts chopped for serving

Directions:

⇒ Put avocados in a kitchen blender and pulse well.

⇒ Add cocoa powder, almond milk, maple syrup, cinnamon and vanilla extract and pulse well again.

⇒ Pour into serving bowls, top with walnuts and keep in the fridge for 2-3 hours before you serve it.

Nutrition: calories 536, fat 36,1, fiber 12,9, carbs 60,7, protein 6,2

99) Dates and Plums Smoothie Bowls

Preparation Time: 2 hours **Cooking Time: 0 minutes** **Servings:4**

Ingredients:

- 1 cup dates, pitted and chopped
- 3 cups plums, chopped
- 2 and ½ cups water
- 1 teaspoon lemon juice

Directions:

⇒ Put dates and plums in a food processor and blend well.

⇒ Add water gradually and pulse a few more times.

⇒ Add lemon juice, pulse for a few more seconds, transfer to a bowl and keep in the freezer for 2 hours.

⇒ Scoop into dessert cups and serve right away!

Nutrition: calories 148, fat 0,3, carbs 39,4, fiber 4,3, protein 1,5

100) Green Avocado Bowls

Preparation Time: 6 minutes **Cooking Time:** **Servings:4**

Ingredients:

- ½ cup coconut water
- 1 and ½ cup avocado, chopped
- 2 tablespoons green tea powder
- 2 teaspoons lime zest
- 1 tablespoon honey
- Melted coconut butter for serving
- 1 mango thinly sliced for serving

Directions:

⇒ In a blender, mix water with avocado, green tea powder and lime zest and pulse well.

⇒ Add honey and pulse again well.

⇒ Transfer to a bowl, top with coconut butter spread all over and serve with sliced mango.

Nutrition: calories 216, fat 15,7, fiber 8,6, carbs 18,4, protein 4,7

101) Maple Ice Cream

Preparation Time: 2 hours **Cooking Time: 3 minutes** **Servings:8**

Ingredients:

- 1 tablespoon arrowroot powder
- 2 cans coconut milk
- ¼ teaspoon vanilla beans
- 1 tablespoon water
- 1/3 cup pure maple syrup
- 1/3 cup coconut nectar

Directions:

⇒ Fill 1/3 of a bowl with ice cubes, place another bowl on top and leave aside for now.

⇒ Pour coconut milk in a saucepan, reserve 2 tablespoons, put them in a bowl, mix with arrowroot starch and stir well.

⇒ Add arrowroot mix of coconut milk to the saucepan and stir.

⇒ Also add vanilla beans, maple syrup and coconut nectar, stir well, place on stove and heat up over medium heat.

⇒ Stir well, bring to a boil, boil for 2 minutes, take off heat and pour into the bowl you've placed over the ice.

⇒ Add water, stir well and leave aside for 1 hour and 30 minutes.

⇒ Pour this into your ice cream machine and turn on.

⇒ Pour into a container, place in the freezer and leave it there for 20 minutes.

⇒ Serve right away!

Nutrition: calories 151, fat 14,5, fiber 1,5, carbs 6, protein 1,4

102) Fruity Cashew Cream

Preparation Time: 6 hours and 10 minutes   **Cooking Time: 0 minutes**   **Servings:6**

Ingredients:

- 1 cup apples, chopped
- 1 cup pineapple, chopped
- 1 cup chickoo, chopped
- 1 cup melon, chopped
- 1 cup papaya, chopped
- ½ teaspoon vanilla powder
- ¾ cup cashews
- Stevia to the taste
- Some cold water

Directions:

⇒ Put cashews in a bowl, add some water on top, leave aside for 6 hours, drain them and put them in a food processor.

⇒ Blend them well and add cold water to cover them.

⇒ Also add stevia and vanilla, blend some more and keep in the fridge for now.

⇒ In a bowl, arrange a layer of mixed apples with pineapples, melon, papaya and chickoo

⇒ Add a layer of cold cashew paste, another layer of fruits, another one of cashew paste and to with a layer of fruits.

⇒ Serve right away!

Nutrition: calories 282, fat 1867, fiber 3,1, carbs 26,5, protein 6,7

103) Chia and Almond Pudding

Preparation Time: 2 hours   **Cooking Time: 0 minutes**   **Servings:4**

Ingredients:

- 2 tablespoons cocoa powder
- 1 cup almond milk
- 1 tablespoon chia seeds
- A pinch of salt
- ½ teaspoon vanilla extract

Directions:

⇒ In a bowl, mix cocoa powder, almond milk, vanilla extract and chia seeds and stir well until they blend.

⇒ Transfer to a dessert glass, place in the fridge for 2 hours and then serve.

Nutrition: calories 180, fat 16,8, fiber 4,7, carbs 7,9, protein 3

104) Matcha Muffins

Preparation Time: 40 minutes   **Cooking Time: 0 minutes**   **Servings:4**

Ingredients:

- 5 tablespoons almond flour
- ½ cup soft coconut butter
- ¾ cup cocoa powder
- ¼ cup cocoa butter
- 1 teaspoon matcha powder (and some more for the topping)
- 3 tablespoons maple syrup
- 1 teaspoon coconut oil
- Cocoa nibs

Directions:

⇒ In a bowl, mix coconut butter with almond flour, maple syrup and matcha powder, stir, cover and keep in the fridge for 10 minutes.

⇒ Put cocoa butter and cocoa powder in a bowl and mix with coconut oil.

⇒ Spoon 2 teaspoons of this melted mix in a muffin liner.

⇒ Repeat this with 7 other muffin liners.

⇒ Take 1 tablespoon matcha mix and shape a ball, place in a muffin liner, press to flatten it and repeat this with the rest of the muffin liners.

⇒ Top each with 1 tablespoon cocoa mass and spread evenly.

⇒ Sprinkle some matcha powder all over muffins.

⇒ Add cocoa nibs on top of each, place them in the freezer and keep there until they are solid.

⇒ Take them out of the freezer, leave at room temperature for a few minutes and serve.

Nutrition: calories 522, fat 46,5, fiber 13,3, carbs 32,4, protein 7,7

105) Almond Ice Cream

Preparation Time: 10 minutes   **Cooking Time: 6 minutes**   Servings:6

Ingredients:

For the caramel sauce:

- ¾ cup stevia
- ½ cup coconut milk
- 2 tablespoons maple syrup
- 1 teaspoon vanilla extract

For the ice cream:

- 12 ounces firm almond cheese
- 1 can coconut milk
- 100 drops liquid stevia
- 2 teaspoons guar

Directions:

⇒ In a pan, heat over medium-high heat ½ cup coconut milk, ¾ cup stevia and maple syrup.

⇒ Stir well, bring to a boil, reduce heat to low and simmer for 3-4 minutes.

⇒ Take off heat, add vanilla extract, stir and leave in the fridge to cool down completely.

⇒ In a food processor, mix coconut milk, almond cheese, a pinch of salt and the caramel and pulse well.

⇒ Add guar and blend again well.

⇒ Take mix from the fridge and transfer to an ice cream maker.

⇒ When the ice cream is done, transfer to bowls and serve with caramel on top.

Nutrition: calories 250, fat 17,6, fiber 0,9, carbs 23,7, protein 7,8

106) Pumpkin Pudding

Preparation Time: 1 hour and 20 minutes   **Cooking Time: 0 minutes**   Servings:4

Ingredients:

- 1 cup almond milk
- ½ cup pumpkin puree
- 2 tablespoons maple syrup
- ½ cup coconut milk

- ½ teaspoon cinnamon powder
- ½ teaspoon vanilla extract
- ¼ teaspoon ginger, grated
- ¼ cup chia seeds

Directions:

⇒ In a bowl, mix almond milk with coconut milk, pumpkin puree, cinnamon, maple syrup, vanilla and ginger and stir well.

⇒ Add chia seeds, stir and leave aside for 20 minutes.

⇒ Divide into 4 glasses, cover and keep in the fridge for 1 hour.

Nutrition: calories 314, fat 25,9, fiber 7,8, carbs 20,3, protein 4,8

107) Cashew Fudge

Preparation Time: 30 minutes   **Cooking Time: 0 minutes**   Servings:4

Ingredients:

- 1/3 cup natural cashew butter
- 1 and ½ tablespoons coconut oil
- 2 tablespoons coconut butter
- 5 tablespoons lemon juice

- ½ teaspoon lemon zest
- A pinch of salt
- 1 tablespoons maple syrup

Directions:

⇒ In a bowl, mix cashew butter with coconut one, coconut oil, lemon juice, lemon zest, a pinch of salt and maple syrup and stir until you obtain a creamy mix.

⇒ Line a muffin tray with some parchment paper, scoop 1 tablespoon of fudge mix in each of the 10 pieces, place in the freezer and keep the for a few hours.

⇒ Take out of the fridge 20 minutes before you serve them.

Nutrition: calories 161, fat 14, fiber 2,9, carbs 11,2, protein 3,7

108) Hemp and Berry Bars

Preparation Time: 30 minutes   **Cooking Time: 0 minutes**   **Servings:6**

Ingredients:

- ¼ cup cocoa nibs
- 1 cup almonds, soaked for at least 3 hours
- 2 tablespoons cocoa powder
- ¼ cup hemp seeds

- ¼ cup goji berries
- ¼ cup coconut, shredded
- 8 dates, pitted and soaked

Directions:

⇒ Put almonds in a food processor and blend them well.

⇒ Add hemp seeds, cocoa nibs, cocoa powder, goji, coconut and blend well.

⇒ Add dates gradually and blend some more.

⇒ Transfer mix to a parchment paper, spread and press it.

⇒ Cut in equal pieces and serve after you've kept them in the fridge for 30 minutes.

Nutrition: calories 304, fat 16,8, fiber 6,1, carbs 32,8, protein 8,4

Chapter 10 - Paleo Gillian's Meal Plan – for Men

Day 1

2) Coconut Berry Smoothie | Calories 222

16) Herbed Chicken and Olives Stew | Calories 553

32) Garlic Potato and Pine Nuts Cream | Calories 445

43) Banana and Walnut Snack | Calories 464

51) Baked Kale Bowls | Calories 9

64) Coffee Steaks | Calories 621

Total Calories 2314

Day 3

7) Coconut Smoothie | Calories 336

23) Chicken, Tomato and Kale Soup | Calories 1227

33) Asparagus and Green Onions Mix | Calories 141

50) Chicken Platter | Calories 485

55) Salsa Pork Mix | Calories 1013

75) Clams and Apple Mix | Calories 610

Total Calories 3812

Day 5

13) Poached Eggs with Artichokes and Lemon Sauce | Calories 1130

19) Nutmeg Coconut and Squash Cream | Calories 245

38) Balsamic Peppers and Capers Mix | Calories 123

45) Thyme Zucchini Fries | Calories 106

58) Balsamic Pork Mix | Calories 271

83) Cayenne Scallops and Avocado Salad | Calories 592

Total Calories 2467

Day 7

8) Walnut and Hemp Bowls | Calories 403

25) Mustard Mushroom Cream | Calories 171

41) Paprika Okra Mix | Calories 107

49) Dehydrated Beef Bites | Calories 273

61) Turkey with Peppers and Tomatoes | Calories 306

87) Lemon Berries and Honeydew Salad | Calories 107

Total Calories 1367

Day 2

3) Lemon Kale Smoothie | Calories 138

19) Nutmeg Coconut and Squash Cream | Calories 245

35) Garlic and Basil Tomatoes | Calories 91

42) Hot Artichoke Bowls | Calories 109

63) Steaks and Pico de Gallo | Calories 285

77) Shrimp and Parsley Mix | Calories 374

Total Calories 1242

Day 4

10) Coconut Orange Bowls | Calories 672

30) Shallot and Cauliflower Cream | Calories 291

40) Lemon Chili Cabbage | Calories 118

48) Coconut Chicken Bites | Calories 330

60) Garlic Pork and Strawberries | Calories 981

90) Chicken and Eggs Salad | Calories 678

Total Calories 3070

Day 6

5) Mint Berry Smoothie | Calories 59

28) Coconut Zucchini Cream | Calories 122

36) Garlic Spinach | Calories 146

47) Turkey Balls | Calories 71

56) Smoked Pork Ribs | Calories 1483

69) Shrimp and Radish Cakes | Calories 406

Total Calories 2287

Chapter 11 -   Conclusion

Always remember to consult with your medical professional before starting any dietary path.

I hope this book can be the springboard to start your long term transformation journey

You can check out (or give away) the other books in the series, just search for Kaylee Gillian.

Regards

Kaylee

Paleo Diet Cookbook on a Budget

Paleo Gillian's Meal Plan| Discover the Nutrition of Our Ancestors Without Spending a Fortune| Delicious Recipes Suitable for Athletes, Men, Women

By Kaylee Gillian

Chapter 1 -   Introduction

Is the Paleo Diet expensive?

The essence of the paleo diet is to eat simply as our hunter-gatherer ancestors did.

Therefore, one should avoid industrially processed foods, refined foods, junk foods, sugary drinks, carbonated drinks etc.

In this book you will discover how easy it is in a paleo diet to save money spent unnecessarily on buying these expensive and unhealthy foods.

Before you leave to go grocery shopping, an idea as simple as taking inventory of foods to buy to fill your pantry will help you conserve your budget.Weekly meal planning and creating a shopping list will help you save money on groceries and gas for cooking.

The recipes in this book will serve to ensure maximum taste, in line with the paleo diet, and are designed to help you save as much as possible on your weekly budget

Enjoy!

Chapter 2 -   Breakfast Recipes

1) Mushroom and Coconut Scramble

Preparation Time: 10 minutes   **Cooking Time: 10 minutes**   **Servings:1**

Ingredients:

- 2 tablespoons ghee, melted
- ¼ cup coconut milk
- 3 eggs

- 3.5 ounces smoked ham, chopped
- 3 ounces mushrooms, sliced
- A pinch of black pepper

Directions:

⇒ Heat up a pan with half of the ghee over medium heat, add the mushrooms, stir and cook for 3 minutes.

⇒ Add ham, stir, cook for 2-3 minutes more and transfer everything to a plate.

⇒ In a bowl, mix eggs with coconut milk and black pepper and whisk.

⇒ Heat up the pan with the rest of the ghee over medium heat, add the eggs, spread into the pan, cook for 5 minutes, stirring often and transfer to a plate.

⇒ Add the mushrooms mix on top, toss a bit and serve.

Nutrition: calories 731, fat 61,7, fiber 3,5, carbs 11, protein 37,2

2) Maple Pancakes

Preparation Time: 10 minutes   **Cooking Time: 10 minutes**   **Servings:8**

Ingredients:

- ¼ cup coconut milk
- ¼ cup coconut flour
- 1/8 teaspoon baking soda
- 3 eggs

- 2 tablespoons coconut oil
- ½ teaspoon vanilla extract
- 2 tablespoons melted ghee

Directions:

⇒ In a bowl, mix the eggs with the coconut oil, vanilla, coconut milk, baking soda and coconut flour and stir very well.

⇒ Heat up a pan with the ghee over medium heat, add 1/8 of the batter, spread into the pan, cook for 2-3 minutes on each side and transfer to a plate

⇒ Repeat with the rest of the batter, divide your pancakes between plates and serve them.

Nutrition: calories 151, fat 10,5, fiber 4,7, carbs 11,4, protein 3,8

3) Cinnamon Almond Pancakes

Preparation Time: 10 minutes   **Cooking Time: 20 minutes**   **Servings:10**

Ingredients:

- 2 cups apples, peeled, cored and chopped
- 1 tablespoon coconut oil, melted
- 4 eggs, whisked
- 2 teaspoons cinnamon powder
- 1 cup almond milk

- 1 teaspoon vanilla extract
- ½ cup coconut flour
- ½ teaspoon baking soda
- 3 tablespoons ghee, melted
- 4 tablespoons maple syrup

Directions:

⇒ Heat up a pan with the oil over medium heat, add the apples and cinnamon, stir and cook for 5 minutes.

⇒ In a bowl, whisk eggs with vanilla, milk, baking soda, coconut flour and the apples and whisk well.

⇒ Heat up a pan with the ghee over medium-high heat, add 1/10 of the batter, spread, cook for 3 minutes on each side and transfer to a plate

⇒ Repeat with the rest of the batter and serve your pancakes with the rest of the maple syrup on top.

Nutrition: calories 213, fat 13,8, fiber 5,8, carbs 20,1, protein 4,3

4) Almond Porridge

Preparation Time: 10 minutes   **Cooking Time: 6 minutes**   **Servings:3**

Ingredients:

- 1 large plantain, peeled and mashed
- ¼ cup flax meal
- 2 cups coconut milk
- ¾ cup almond meal

- 1 teaspoon cinnamon, powder
- A pinch of cloves, ground
- ½ teaspoon ginger powder
- A pinch of nutmeg, ground

Directions:

⇒ In a small saucepan, mix all the ingredients, bring to a simmer and cook for 6 minutes.

⇒ Divide the porridge into bowls and serve.

Nutrition: calories 622, fat 53,7, fiber 11, carbs 36,6, protein 11,5

5) Walnuts Porridge

Preparation Time: 10 minutes   **Cooking Time: 5 minutes**   **Servings:2**

Ingredients:

- ½ cup walnuts, soaked overnight and drained
- 1 banana, peeled and mashed
- ¾ cup hot water

- 2 tablespoons coconut butter
- ½ teaspoon cinnamon powder

Directions:

⇒ In a blender, mix all the ingredients, pulse well and transfer to a saucepan.

⇒ Heat everything over medium heat, cook for 5 minutes, transfer to bowls and serve.

Nutrition: calories 353, fat 28,6, fiber 3,7, carbs 21,1, protein 8,2

6) Turkey Stuffed Mushroom Caps

Preparation Time: 5 minutes   **Cooking Time: 10 minutes**   **Servings:1**

Ingredients:

- 2 Portobello mushroom caps
- 2 lettuce leaves
- 2 avocado slices

- ½ pound turkey meat, cooked, sliced
- Olive oil

Directions:

⇒ Heat up a pan over medium-high heat, add the turkey meat, cook for 4 minutes, transfer to paper towels to drain excess oil.

⇒ Heat up the pan with the olive oil over medium high heat, add mushroom caps, cook for 2 minutes on each side and take off heat.

⇒ Arrange 1 mushroom cap on a plate, add turkey, avocado slices, and lettuce leaves, top with the other mushroom cap and serve.

Nutrition: calories 521, fat 25,5, fiber 0,9, carbs 3,1, protein 67,9

7) Turkey and Egg Sandwich

Preparation Time: 5 minutes   **Cooking Time: 10 minutes**   **Servings:2**

Ingredients:

- 2 cups bell peppers, chopped
- ½ tablespoon avocado oil
- 3 eggs

- 15 oz turkey fillet, cooked, sliced
- Olive oil

Directions:

⇒ Heat up a pan with the oil over medium-high heat, add bell peppers, stir and cook for 5 minutes

⇒ Heat up another pan over medium heat, add the turkey meat, stir, cook for 3-4 minutes, drain excess oil and transfer to a bowl,

⇒ In a bowl, whisk the eggs well, add them to the pan with the bell peppers, stir and cook for 7-8 minutes.

⇒ Divide half of the turkey slices between plates, add eggs, top with the other turkey slices and serve.

Nutrition: calories 580, fat 25,6, fiber 1,8, carbs 9,7, protein 75,4

8) Stuffed Mushrooms

Preparation Time: 10 minutes **Cooking Time: 15 minutes** **Servings:3**

Ingredients:

- 3 Portobello mushroom caps
- 10 oz turkey meat, cooked, sliced
- 3 eggs
- 4 ounces smoked salmon
- Olive oil

Directions:

⇒ Heat up a pan over medium-high heat, add the turkey, cook for 4 minutes, transfer to paper towels to drain excess oil.

⇒ Heat up the pan with the olive oil over medium heat, place egg rings in the pan, crack an egg in each, cook them for 6 minutes and transfer them to a plate.

⇒ Heat up the pan again over medium-high heat, add mushroom caps, cook for 5 minutes and transfer them to a platter.

⇒ Top each mushroom cap with turkey slices, salmon, and eggs and serve.

Nutrition: calories 315, fat 15,5, fiber 0,4, carbs 1,8, protein 40,8

9) Veggie and Beef Pan

Preparation Time: 10 minutes **Cooking Time: 20 minutes** **Servings:3**

Ingredients:

- 15 ounces beef, ground
- 2 tablespoons ghee
- 3 garlic cloves, minced
- 2 celery stalks, chopped
- 1 yellow onion, chopped
- A pinch of sea salt and black pepper
- ½ teaspoon coriander, ground
- 1 teaspoon cumin, ground
- 1 teaspoon garam masala
- ½ butternut squash, chopped and already cooked
- 3 eggs, whisked
- 1 small avocado, peeled, pitted and chopped
- 15 ounces spinach, torn

Directions:

⇒ Heat up a pan with the ghee over medium heat, add onion, garlic, celery, a pinch of salt and pepper, stir and cook for 3 minutes.

⇒ Add beef, cumin, garam masala, and coriander, stir and cook for 5 minutes more.

⇒ Add squash flesh and spinach, stir and make 3 holes in this mix.

⇒ Crack an egg into each, cover the pan, place in the oven at 375 degrees F, bake for 15 minutes, divide between plates and serve with avocado on top.

Nutrition: calories 594, fat 35,6, fiber 9,2, carbs 19, protein 54,9

10) Turkey and Eggs Pan

Preparation Time: 10 minutes **Cooking Time: 15 minutes** **Servings:4**

Ingredients:

- 20 ounces turkey meat, cooked, ground
- 4 tablespoons coconut oil
- 1 small green bell pepper, chopped
- ½ cup onion, chopped
- 2 garlic cloves, minced
- 2 cups sweet potato, chopped
- 1 avocado, peeled, pitted, cut into halves and thinly sliced
- 3 eggs
- 2 cups spinach

Directions:

⇒ Heat up a pan with the oil over medium-high heat, add onion, stir and cook for 3 minutes.

⇒ Add garlic and bell pepper, stir and cook for 1 minute.

⇒ Add the ground turkey, stir and brown for 15 minutes more.

⇒ Add sweet potato, stir and cook for 4 minutes.

⇒ Add spinach, stir and cook for 2 minutes.

⇒ Make 3 holes in this mix, crack an egg in each, place pan under a preheated broiler and cook for 3 minutes.

⇒ Divide between plates, top with avocado slices and serve.

Nutrition: calories 619, fat 34,1, fiber 7,8, carbs 29,9, protein 49,6

Chapter 3 -   Soup & Stew Recipes

11) Sweet Potato, Tomato and Beef Stew

Preparation Time: 10 minutes   **Cooking Time: 35 minutes**   **Servings:4**

Ingredients:

- 1 red onion, chopped
- 1 tablespoon balsamic vinegar
- 2 tablespoons coconut oil, melted
- A pinch of sea salt and black pepper
- 1 pound beef, ground
- 3 garlic cloves, minced
- 2/3 teaspoon ginger, grated
- 1 teaspoon coriander seeds
- 1 teaspoon cumin, ground
- 1 teaspoon sweet paprika
- 3 cups sweet potatoes, peeled and cubed
- 1 and ½ cups veggie stock
- 1 carrot, chopped
- 10 oz fresh tomatoes, peeled, chopped
- ¼ cup parsley, chopped
- Zest of 1 lemon, grated

Directions:

⇒ Heat up a large saucepan with the oil over medium heat, add the onion, stir and sauté for 10 minutes.

⇒ Add vinegar, stir and cook for 1 minute more.

⇒ Add ginger and the meat, stir and cook for 2 minutes.

⇒ Add garlic, coriander, cumin, and paprika, stir and cook for 2 minutes.

⇒ Add stock, carrot, tomatoes and lemon zest, stir, cover and cook for 20 minutes.

⇒ Add parsley, stir, cook for 2 minutes more, divide into bowls and serve.

Nutrition: calories 455, fat 17, fiber 6,9, carbs 42,5, protein 37,6

12) Garlic Chicken Stew

Preparation Time: 10 minutes   **Cooking Time: 8 hours**   **Servings:6**

Ingredients:

- 2 carrots, chopped
- 5 garlic cloves, minced
- 2 celery sticks, chopped
- 2 yellow onions, chopped
- 2 sweet potatoes, cubed
- 25 ounces homemade pumpkin puree
- 2 cups chicken stock
- 2 cups chicken meat, skinless, boneless and shredded
- A pinch of sea salt and black pepper
- ¼ teaspoon cayenne pepper

Directions:

⇒ In a slow cooker, combine all the ingredients, toss, cover and cook on Low for 8 hours.

⇒ Divide into bowls and serve.

Nutrition: calories 230, fat 3,8, fiber 6,6, carbs 31,9, protein 17,3

13) Thyme Beef Stew

Preparation Time: 10 minutes   **Cooking Time: 7 hours and 10 minutes**   **Servings:4**

Ingredients:

- 2 tablespoons olive oil
- 8 carrots, chopped
- 2 parsnips, chopped
- 1 and ½ pounds beef meat, cubed
- ½ teaspoon peppercorns
- 1 yellow onion, chopped
- 1 tablespoon thyme, chopped
- 2 tablespoons water
- 4 cups beef stock
- A pinch of sea salt and black pepper

Directions:

⇒ Heat up a large saucepan with the oil over medium-high heat, add the beef, stir, brown for 4 minutes on all sides and transfer to your slow cooker.

⇒ Add all the other ingredients, cover and cook on Low for 7 hours.

⇒ Divide the stew into bowls and serve.

Nutrition: calories 575, fat 23,8, fiber 5,5, carbs 21,3, protein 66,5

14) Baharat Stew

Preparation Time: 10 minutes   **Cooking Time: 8 hours**   **Servings:6**

Ingredients:

- 1 cup carrots, chopped
- 1 cup celery, chopped
- 2 cups onions, chopped
- 3 pounds osso buco, bones in
- 4 garlic cloves, minced
- 6 teaspoons baharat
- A pinch of black pepper
- 2 cups beef stock
- A handful parsley, chopped
- 1 kale, chopped

Directions:

⇒ In a slow cooker, combine all the ingredients except the kale and the parsley, toss, cover and cook on Low for 7 hours and 30 minutes.

⇒ Add the kale, cook the stew on Low for 30 minutes more, divide into bowls, sprinkle the parsley on top and serve.

Nutrition: Calories 291, fat 7,9, fiber 1,7, carbs 7,1, protein 42,8

15) Lamb and Celery Stew

Preparation Time: 10 minutes   **Cooking Time: 2 hours**   **Servings:4**

Ingredients:

- 1 and ½ pounds lamb meat, cubed
- 1 tablespoon olive oil
- 1 small red chili pepper, chopped
- 1 yellow onion, chopped
- 3 garlic cloves, minced
- 2 celery sticks, chopped
- 2 and ½ teaspoons garam masala
- 1 and ¼ teaspoons turmeric powder
- 1 and ½ cups coconut milk
- 1 and ½ teaspoons ghee
- 1 and ½ tablespoons tomato paste
- 2 carrots, chopped
- 1 cup water
- A pinch of sea salt and black pepper
- 1 tablespoon lemon juice
- 1 tablespoon cilantro, chopped

Directions:

⇒ Heat up a large saucepan with the oil over medium-high heat, add the lamb, and brown for 4 minutes on all sides.

⇒ Add celery, chili and onion, stir and cook for 1 minute.

⇒ Reduce the heat to medium, add turmeric, garam masala, garlic and the ghee, stir and cook for 2 minutes more.

⇒ Add tomato paste, coconut milk, water, salt and pepper, stir, bring to a boil, cover and cook for 1 hour.

⇒ Add carrots, stir, cover saucepan again and cook for 40 minutes more.

⇒ Add lemon juice and parsley, stir, divide into bowls and serve hot.

Nutrition: calories 510, fat 32,8, fiber 6,5, carbs 25,9, protein 27,3

16) Tomato and Turnip Stew

Preparation Time: 10 minutes   **Cooking Time: 1 hour**   **Servings:6**

Ingredients:

- 1 garlic head, cloves peeled
- 2 pounds turnips, cubed
- ½ cup yellow onion, chopped
- 6 tablespoons olive oil
- 1 tablespoon tomato paste
- 25 ounces fresh tomatoes, peeled, chopped
- A pinch of sea salt and black pepper
- 2 cups kale, chopped
- 1 teaspoon oregano, dried

Directions:

⇒ In a large baking dish, mix the turnips with garlic cloves, half of the oil, salt and pepper, toss to coat, and bake at 450 degrees F for 45 minutes.

⇒ Heat up a pan with the rest of the oil over medium-high heat, add the onion, stir and cook for 3 minutes.

⇒ Add tomato paste, stir and cook for 1 minute.

⇒ Add tomatoes, oregano, salt and pepper, stir, bring to a simmer and cook for 10 minutes.

⇒ Add the parsnips, and the kale, cook the stew for 5 more minutes, divide into bowls and serve.

Nutrition: calories 208, fat 14,3, fiber 4,7, carbs 19,6, protein 3,4

17) Basil Chicken and Tomato Stew

Preparation Time: 10 minutes **Cooking Time: 2 hours** **Servings:4**

Ingredients:

- 5 garlic cloves, minced
- 2 pounds chicken thighs, skinless, boneless and cubed
- 25 ounces fresh tomatoes, peeled, chopped
- 30 black olives, pitted and chopped
- 2 cups chicken stock
- 2 tablespoons parsley, chopped

- 2 tablespoons thyme, chopped
- 2 tablespoons basil, chopped
- 2 tablespoons coconut oil, melted
- A pinch of sea salt and black pepper
- 2 tablespoons rosemary, chopped

Directions:

⇒ Heat up a large saucepan with the oil over medium-high heat, add chicken pieces, salt and pepper, stir and brown them for 2 minutes on each side.

⇒ Add all the other ingredients, stir, cover, place in the oven at 325 degrees F and bake for 2 hours.

⇒ Divide into bowls and serve.

Nutrition: calories 580, fat 28,2, fiber 4,6, carbs 12,7, protein 68,3

18) Chicken and Onion Stew

Preparation Time: 10 minutes **Cooking Time: 45 minutes** **Servings:4**

Ingredients:

- 4 chicken thighs
- 1 small brown onion, chopped
- ½ tablespoon coconut oil, melted
- A pinch of sea salt and black pepper
- 1 tablespoon ginger, grated
- 1 tablespoon garlic, minced
- ½ teaspoon sweet paprika

- ½ tablespoon coriander
- ½ teaspoon chili powder
- 20 ounces fresh tomatoes, peeled, chopped
- 2 and ½ tablespoons coconut butter, softened
- ¼ cup water
- 1 tablespoon parsley, chopped
- ¼ teaspoon vanilla extract

Directions:

⇒ Heat up a pan with the oil over medium-high heat, add chicken pieces, some salt and black pepper, stir, brown for 4 minutes on each side and transfer them to a bowl.

⇒ Heat the same pan over medium heat, add ginger and onion, stir and sauté for 6 minutes.

⇒ Add garlic, paprika, coriander and chili powder, stir and cook for 1 minute.

⇒ Add water, tomatoes and return the chicken pieces, stir, cover, bring to a boil and simmer for 25 minutes.

⇒ Add the coconut butter and vanilla, stir and cook for 2 minutes more.

⇒ Divide the stew into bowls, sprinkle parsley and serve hot.

Nutrition: calories 1161, fat 98, fiber 26,1, carbs 37,3, protein 39,3

19) Beef and Carrots Stew

Preparation Time: 10 minutes **Cooking Time: 6 hours** **Servings:8**

Ingredients:

- 2 pounds beef stew meat, cubed
- 2 celery stick, chopped
- 2 leeks, chopped
- A pinch of sea salt and black pepper
- 2 tablespoons avocado oil
- 3 thyme springs, chopped

- 4 carrots, chopped
- 3 rosemary springs, chopped
- 2 tablespoons coconut flour
- 25 ounces fresh tomatoes, peeled, chopped
- 1-quart beef stock

Directions:

⇒ In a slow cooker, combine all the ingredients except the flour, cover and cook on High for 5 hours and 30 minutes.

⇒ In a bowl, mix the coconut flour with 2-3 tablespoons liquid from the pot, whisk and add to the slow cooker.

⇒ Cook the stew on Low for 30 minutes more, divide into bowls and serve.

Nutrition: calories 569, fat 16,9, fiber 8,5, carbs 26, protein 75,7

20) Lemongrass Carrots Stew

Preparation Time: 30 minutes **Cooking Time: 3 hours** **Servings:6**

Ingredients:

- 1 lemongrass stalk, chopped
- 2 and ½ pounds organic beef brisket, cubed
- 1 and ½ teaspoons curry powder
- 2 and ½ tablespoons ginger, grated
- 3 tablespoons ghee, melted
- 1 yellow onion, chopped

- 20 ounces fresh tomatoes, peeled, chopped
- 3 cups water
- 1 pound carrots, chopped
- ¼ cup cilantro, chopped
- A pinch of sea salt and black pepper

Directions:

⇒ In a bowl, mix the lemongrass with curry powder, ginger and beef, toss to coat well and leave aside for 30 minutes.

⇒ Heat up a large saucepan with the ghee over medium high heat, add the beef, brown on all sides for 4 minutes and transfer to a plate.

⇒ Return saucepan to medium heat, add the onion, stir and cook for 2 minutes.

⇒ Add salt, black pepper and tomatoes, stir and cook for 15 minutes.

⇒ Return the beef, stir and cook for 5 minutes.

⇒ Add carrots and water, stir, bring to a boil, cover, place in the oven at 300 degrees and bake for 2 hours and 30 minutes.

⇒ Stir the stew, divide into bowls, sprinkle cilantro on top and serve.

Nutrition: calories 551, fat 21,5, fiber 3,5, carbs 13,7, protein 72,4

21) Cumin Eggplant Stew

Preparation Time: 10 minutes **Cooking Time: 25 minutes** **Servings:3**

Ingredients:

- 2 big tomatoes, chopped
- 1 eggplant, chopped
- 1 cup tomato paste
- 1 yellow onion, chopped

- 1 teaspoon cumin powder
- A pinch of salt and cayenne pepper
- ½ cup water

Directions:

⇒ Put the water in a small saucepan, heat up over medium heat, add all the ingredients, toss, bring to a boil and simmer for 25 minutes.

⇒ Divide into bowls and serve.

Nutrition: calories 149, fat 1,1, fiber 11,3, carbs 33,9, protein 6,9

22) Garlic Tomato and Turkey Soup

Preparation Time: 15 minutes   **Cooking Time: 40 minutes**   **Servings:6**

Ingredients:

- 1 yellow onion, chopped
- 1 tablespoon avocado oil
- 3 thyme springs, chopped
- 3 garlic cloves, finely minced
- 25 oz fresh tomatoes, peeled, chopped
- 6 ounces tomato paste

- ¼ cup water
- 1 pound turkey meat, ground, fried
- 14 ounces beef stock
- 6 mushrooms, chopped
- 1 small red bell pepper, chopped
- ½ cup black olives, chopped

Directions:

⇒ Heat a saucepan with the oil over medium-high heat, add half of the onion, garlic and thyme. Stir and cook for 5 minutes.

⇒ Add tomatoes, tomato paste and the water, stir, bring to a boil, reduce heat to medium-low and simmer for 20 minutes.

⇒ Pour this mixture into a blender and pulse well.

⇒ Heat up a saucepan over medium-high heat, add the turkey, stir and cook for 4 minutes, breaking it into small pieces with a fork.

⇒ Add the rest of the onion, mushrooms and the bell pepper, stir and cook for 5 minutes.

⇒ Add blended soup and beef stock, stir and cook for 5 more minutes.

⇒ Ladle the soup into bowls, top with the olives and serve.

Nutrition: calories 218, fat 6, fiber 4,6, carbs 16,3, protein 18,3

23) Coconut Tomato Cream Soup

Preparation Time: 10 minutes   **Cooking Time: 35 minutes**   **Servings:4**

Ingredients:

- 56 oz fresh tomatoes, peeled, crushed
- 2 cups tomato juice
- 2 cups chicken stock
- ¼ pound coconut butter, melted

- 14 basil leaves, torn
- 1 cup coconut milk
- Salt and black pepper to the taste

Directions:

⇒ Put tomatoes, tomato juice and stock in a saucepan, heat up over medium-high heat, bring to a boil, reduce heat, stir and simmer for 30 minutes.

⇒ Pour this into a blender, add basil, pulse very well and return to saucepan.

⇒ Heat up the soup again, add the butter, salt, pepper and coconut milk, stir, cook over low heat for 4 minutes more, divide into bowls and serve.

Nutrition: calories 421, fat 33,5, fiber 11,6, carbs 31,3, protein 8,2

24) Rosemary Chicken Soup

Preparation Time: 15 minutes   **Cooking Time: 60 minutes**   **Servings:4**

Ingredients:

- 2 teaspoons coconut oil, melted
- 3 carrots, chopped
- 1 yellow onion, chopped
- 1 zucchini, chopped
- 15 ounces mushrooms, chopped
- 4 cups chicken meat, already cooked and shredded

- 2 teaspoons rosemary, dried
- 1 teaspoon thyme, dried
- 1 tablespoon apple cider vinegar
- 1 teaspoon cumin, ground
- 2 and ½ cups chicken stock
- A pinch of sea salt and black pepper

Directions:

⇒ Heat up a saucepan with the oil over medium heat, add carrots and onion, stir and cook for 5 minutes.

⇒ Add zucchini, and mushrooms, stir and cook for 10 more minutes.

⇒ Add the chicken meat, rosemary, thyme, vinegar, cumin and the stock, stir, bring to a boil, reduce heat to medium-low and simmer for 40 minutes.

⇒ Add salt and pepper to the taste, stir again, ladle into bowls and serve.

Nutrition: calories 459, fat 16,9, carbs 23,6, protein 52,8, fiber 3,7

25) Turmeric Cauliflower Cream

Preparation Time: 10 minutes   **Cooking Time: 60 minutes**   **Servings:6**

Ingredients:

- 1 yellow onion, chopped
- 2 tablespoons extra virgin olive oil
- 2 pounds cauliflower florets
- A pinch of sea salt and black pepper
- ½ teaspoon turmeric powder
- 2 garlic cloves, minced
- 5 cups veggie stock

Directions:

⇒ Heat up a saucepan with the oil over medium heat, add the onion and garlic, stir and sauté for 10 minutes.

⇒ Add cauliflower, salt and pepper, stir and cook for 12 more minutes.

⇒ Add the stock, stir, bring to a boil, reduce heat to medium and simmer for 25 minutes.

⇒ Transfer to a blender, add the turmeric powder, pulse well, ladle into bowls and serve.

Nutrition: calories 100, fat 6,8, carbs 12,4, fiber 4,3, protein 3,3

Chapter 4 - Side Recipes

26) Spinach and Pumpkin Mix

Preparation Time: 10 minutes **Cooking Time: 30 minutes** **Servings:6**

Ingredients:

- 2 tablespoons olive oil + 2 teaspoons olive oil
- 21 ounces pumpkin, peeled, seeded and cubed
- 2 teaspoons sesame seeds
- 1 tablespoon lemon juice

- 2 teaspoons mustard
- 4 ounces baby spinach
- 2 tablespoons pine nuts, toasted
- A pinch of sea salt and black pepper

Directions:

⇒ In a bowl, mix pumpkin with salt, black pepper and 2 teaspoons oil, toss to coat well, spread on a lined baking sheet, place in the oven at 400 degrees F and bake for 25 minutes.

⇒ Leave pumpkin pieces to cool down a bit, add sesame seeds, toss to coat, place in the oven again and bake for 5 minutes more.

⇒ In a bowl, mix lemon juice with the rest of the oil and mustard and whisk.

⇒ Leave pumpkin to completely cool down and transfer it to a salad bowl.

⇒ Add baby spinach, pine nuts and the salad dressing, toss to coat well, divide between plates and serve as a side salad.

Nutrition: calories 149, fat 12,5, fiber 3,7, carbs 9,8, protein 2,5

27) Rosemary Turnips

Preparation Time: 10 minutes **Cooking Time: 15 minutes** **Servings:4**

Ingredients:

- 1 tablespoon lemon juice
- Zest of 2 oranges
- 16 ounces turnips, thinly sliced
- 3 tablespoons coconut oil

- 1 tablespoon rosemary, chopped
- A pinch of sea salt
- Black pepper to taste

Directions:

⇒ Heat up a pan with the oil over medium-high heat, add turnips, stir and cook for 4 minutes.

⇒ Add lemon juice, a pinch of salt, black pepper, and rosemary, stir and cook for 10 minutes more.

⇒ Take off the heat, add orange zest, stir, divide between plates and serve.

Nutrition: calories 125, fat 10,4, fiber 2,3, carbs 8,2, protein 1

28) Fennel Salad

Preparation Time: 10 minutes **Cooking Time: 0 minutes** **Servings:4**

Ingredients:

- 3 tablespoons lemon juice
- 1-pound fennel, chopped

- A pinch of sea salt and black pepper
- 2 tablespoons olive oil

Directions:

⇒ In a salad bowl, mix fennel with a pinch of salt and black pepper and toss,

⇒ In another bowl, mix the oil with a pinch of salt, pepper and lemon juice and whisk well.

⇒ Add this to the salad bowl, toss to coat well, divide between plates and serve as a side dish.

Nutrition: calories 98, fat 7,3, fiber 3,6, carbs 8,5, protein 1,5

29) Fried Green Plantains

Preparation Time: 10 minutes   **Cooking Time: 10 minutes**   **Servings:4**

Ingredients:

- ½ cup ghee, melted
- 2 green plantains, peeled and sliced
- A pinch of sea salt and black pepper

Directions:

⇒ Heat up a pan with the ghee over medium-high heat, season plantain slices with salt and black pepper, add half of them to the pan, cook for 5 minutes and transfer to paper towels.

⇒ Fry the second batch of plantain slices, drain grease as well, divide them between plates and serve them as a side.

Nutrition: calories 334, fat 25,8, fiber 2,1, carbs 28,5, protein 1,2

30) Garlic Broccoli

Preparation Time: 10 minutes   **Cooking Time: 30 minutes**   **Servings:4**

Ingredients:

- 8 garlic cloves, minced
- ¼ cup avocado oil
- 8 cups broccoli florets
- Zest of 1 lemon, grated
- ¼ cup parsley, chopped
- A pinch of sea salt and black pepper

Directions:

⇒ In a bowl, mix broccoli with salt, pepper, oil, garlic and lemon zest, toss to coat, spread on a lined baking sheet, place in the oven at 450 degrees F and bake for 30 minutes.

⇒ Divide between plates, sprinkle parsley on top and serve as a side.

Nutrition: calories 92, fat 2,4, fiber 5,6, carbs 15,1, protein 5,8

31) Kale Salad

Preparation Time: 10 minutes   **Cooking Time: 0 minutes**   **Servings:2**

Ingredients:

- 2 cups arugula leaves
- 1 tablespoon olive oil
- 1 tablespoon balsamic vinegar
- 2 cups kale, torn
- 3 tablespoons red onion, chopped
- 4 kumquats, sliced
- 1 small avocado, pitted, peeled and cubed
- ½ cup walnuts, chopped

Directions:

⇒ In a bowl, combine all the ingredients, toss, divide between plates and serve as a side dish.

Nutrition: calories 531, fat 45,5, fiber 13, carbs 27, protein 12,8

32) Simple Sprouts Mix

Preparation Time: 10 minutes   **Cooking Time: 30 minutes**   **Servings:4**

Ingredients:

- ¼ cup avocado oil
- 4 pounds Brussels sprouts, halved
- A pinch of sea salt and black pepper

Directions:

⇒ In a bowl, mix Brussels sprouts with oil, salt, and pepper, toss to coat well, spread on a lined baking sheet, place in the oven at 375 degrees F and bake for 30 minutes.

⇒ Divide between plates and serve as a side dish.

Nutrition: calories 215, fat 3,3, fiber 17,6, carbs 42, protein 15,6

33) Baked Squash Mix

Preparation Time: 10 minutes   **Cooking Time: 1 hour and 30 minutes**   **Servings:8**

Ingredients:

- 1 pound yellow squash, peeled and chopped
- 1 yellow onion, chopped
- 3 tablespoons olive oil
- 2 garlic cloves, minced

- 4 pounds mixed sweet potatoes, cubed
- 1 cup veggie stock
- A pinch of black pepper

Directions:

⇒ In a baking dish, combine all the ingredients, toss and bake at 400 degrees F and bake for 1 hour.

⇒ Divide between plates and serve warm as a side dish.

Nutrition: calories 555, fat 6,2, fiber 17,5, carbs 120,5, protein 7,2

34) Fried Tapioca Root

Preparation Time: 10 minutes   **Cooking Time: 1 hour**   **Servings:4**

Ingredients:

- 2 and ½ pound tapioca root, cut in medium fries
- ½ cup ghee, melted

- Black pepper to taste

Directions:

⇒ Put some water in a large saucepan, bring to a boil over medium high heat, add tapioca fries, boil for 10 minutes and drain them well.

⇒ Spread the fries on a lined baking sheet, add black pepper and the ghee, toss everything to coat well, place in the oven at 375 degrees F and bake for 45 minutes.

⇒ Divide them between plates and serve as a side.

Nutrition: calories 905, fat 25,5, fiber 1,7, carbs 168,5, protein 0,4

35) Baked Cauliflower

Preparation Time: 10 minutes   **Cooking Time: 30 minutes**   **Servings:4**

Ingredients:

- 6 cups cauliflower florets
- 1 and ½ pounds turnips, thinly sliced
- 1 cup chicken stock

- 2 tablespoons avocado oil
- A pinch of sea salt and black pepper

Directions:

⇒ In a baking dish, toss well to combine all the ingredients, and bake at 375 degrees F for 30 minutes.

⇒ Divide between plates and serve.

Nutrition: calories 140, fat 1,5, fiber 9,9, carbs 29,4, protein 6,2

Chapter 5 -   Snack & Appetizer Recipes

36) Hot Pepper Chips

Preparation Time: 10 minutes   **Cooking Time: 13 minutes**   **Servings:4**

Ingredients:

- 10 shishito peppers
- Juice of ½ lemon
- 2 teaspoons olive oil
- 1 garlic clove, minced
- A pinch of sea salt
- Black pepper to taste

Directions:

⇒ Heat up a pan with the oil over medium high heat, add peppers, lemon juice, garlic, a pinch of salt and black pepper, stir and cook for 10 minutes.

⇒ Drain excess grease on paper towels, arrange on a small platter and serve.

Nutrition: calories 62, fat 2,4, fiber 5,1, carbs 8,8, protein 2,6

37) Potato Balls

Preparation Time: 10 minutes   **Cooking Time: 25 minutes**   **Servings:18**

Ingredients:

- 2 cups sweet potatoes, peeled, cubed and boiled
- 2 garlic cloves, minced
- 4 tablespoons cilantro, chopped
- 1 teaspoon black pepper
- A pinch of sea salt
- Juice of 2 limes
- A pinch of cayenne pepper
- 2 tablespoons nutritional yeast

Directions:

⇒ In a bowl mix sweet potatoes with a pinch of salt and pepper and mash well.

⇒ Add garlic, cilantro, a black pepper, lime juice, cayenne and nutritional yeast and stir very well.

⇒ Shape small balls out of this mix, arrange them on a baking sheet, place in the oven at 350 degrees F and bake for 25 minutes.

⇒ Arrange balls on a platter and serve them cold.

Nutrition: calories 25, fat 0,1, fiber 1, carbs 5,7, protein 0,8

38) Chicken Platter

Preparation Time: 10 minutes   **Cooking Time: 45 minutes**   **Servings:13**

Ingredients:

- 2 pounds chicken breasts, skinless, boneless and cubed
- 1 adobo chili pepper, chopped
- ¼ cup tomato sauce

Directions:

⇒ Put the tomato sauce in a large saucepan, heat up over medium heat, add the chili, stir and bring to a boil.

⇒ Add the chicken cubes, toss, spread on a lined baking sheet, and bake at 375 degrees F and bake for 45 minutes.

⇒ Leave chicken bites to cool down, arrange them on a platter and serve.

Nutrition: calories 135, fat 5,2, fiber 0,1, carbs 0,6, protein 20,3

39) Turkey and Scallops Platter

Preparation Time: 10 minutes   **Cooking Time: 16 minutes**   **Servings:4**

Ingredients:

- 20 sea scallops
- 5 ounces turkey meat, cooked, sliced
- ½ cup baby spinach leaves
- ¼ cup red onion, chopped
- ½ teaspoon curry powder
- ½ teaspoon red pepper, ground
- A pinch of sea salt

- 1 tablespoon coconut oil

  For the sauce:
- 4 tablespoons balsamic vinegar
- 2 shallots, chopped
- ¼ teaspoon coconut sugar
- 1 tablespoon olive oil

Directions:

⇒ Heat up a pan with 1 tablespoon oil over medium-high heat, add turkey, stir, cook until it browns, transfer to paper towels to drain excess grease, cut into medium pieces and leave aside.

⇒ In a bowl, mix red pepper with curry powder and a pinch of sea salt and stir.

⇒ Add scallops and rub them well.

⇒ Heat up the same pan where you cooked the turkey over medium-high heat, sprinkle some olive oil, add scallops and cook them for 3 minutes on each side.

⇒ Heat up the same pan with 1 tablespoon olive oil over medium-high heat, add shallots, stir and cook them for 2 minutes.

⇒ Add the sugar and vinegar, stir, cook until everything thickens and take off heat.

⇒ Arrange turkey meat pieces on a platter, add spinach leaves and onion pieces.

⇒ Top with scallops, stick a toothpick in the middle of each and drizzle the sauce you've made on top.

Nutrition: calories 274, fat 9,9, fiber 0,5, carbs 8,1, protein 36,2

40) Mixed Cabbage Snack

Preparation Time: 10 minutes   **Cooking Time: 2 hours**   **Servings:8**

Ingredients:

- ½ red cabbage head, leaves separated and halved
- ½ green cabbage head, leaves separated and halved
- A drizzle of olive oil

- Black pepper to taste
- A pinch of sea salt

Directions:

⇒ Spread cabbage leaves on a lined baking sheet, place in the oven at 200 degrees F and bake for 2 hours.

⇒ Drizzle the oil over them, sprinkle salt and black pepper, rub well, transfer to a bowl and serve as a snack.

Nutrition: calories 39, fat 0,2, fiber 3,9, carbs 9,1, protein 2

41) Chives Cauliflower Bites

Preparation Time: 5 minutes   **Cooking Time: 30 minutes**   **Servings:1**

Ingredients:

- 1 small cauliflower head, chopped
- A pinch of sea salt
- ½ teaspoon chives, dried

- ½ teaspoon onion powder
- A drizzle of avocado oil

Directions:

⇒ In a bowl, mix cauliflower popcorn with a pinch of salt and the oil, toss to coat, spread them on a lined baking sheet, and bake at 450 degrees F for 30 minutes, tossing the popcorn halfway.

⇒ Transfer the popcorn to a bowl, add chives and onion powder, stir and serve them.

Nutrition: calories 194, fat 14,3, fiber 6,7, carbs 15, protein 5,4

42) Lemon Cashew Spread

Preparation Time: 10 minutes   **Cooking Time: 0 minutes**   **Servings:6**

Ingredients:

- ½ cup cashews, soaked for 2 hours and drained
- 1 tablespoon olive oil
- 2 tablespoons lemon juice
- ½ cup pumpkin puree
- 2 tablespoons sesame paste
- 1 garlic clove, minced
- ¼ teaspoon cumin, ground
- A pinch of cayenne pepper
- A pinch of sea salt
- ½ teaspoon pumpkin spice

Directions:

⇒ In your food processor, mix soaked cashews with lemon juice, pumpkin puree, sesame paste, garlic, cumin, pepper, sea salt and pumpkin spice and blend well.

⇒ Add oil gradually, blend again well, transfer to a bowl and serve as a snack.

Nutrition: calories 99, fat 8,2, fiber 1, carbs 5,7, protein 2,2

43) Avocado Dip

Preparation Time: 10 minutes   **Cooking Time: 0 minutes**   **Servings:4**

Ingredients:

- 3 green onions, chopped
- 3 avocados, pitted, peeled and roughly chopped
- A pinch of pink salt
- 1 teaspoon garlic powder
- Juice of 1 lime

Directions:

⇒ In food processor mix onions with avocados, garlic powder, salt and lime juice and pulse a few times.

⇒ Transfer to a bowl and serve as a snack.

Nutrition: calories 316, fat 29,4, fiber 10,5, carbs 15,2, protein 3,2

44) Lemon Cauliflower Dip

Preparation Time: 10 minutes   **Cooking Time: 40 minutes**   **Servings:4**

Ingredients:

- 4 tablespoons sesame seeds paste
- 1 cauliflower head, florets separated
- 1 small red bell pepper, chopped
- 5 tablespoons olive oil
- 4 tablespoons lemon juice
- 1 teaspoon garlic powder
- Black pepper to taste
- ½ teaspoon cumin, ground
- A pinch of paprika for serving
- A pinch of sea salt

Directions:

⇒ Arrange the cauliflower and bell pepper pieces on a lined baking sheet, drizzle 1 tablespoon over them, toss to coat and bake in the oven at 400 degrees F for 40 minutes.

⇒ Transfer the veggies to a blender, add sesame seeds paste, salt, pepper, the rest of the oil, garlic powder, cumin and lemon juice and blend until you obtain a paste.

⇒ Transfer to a bowl, sprinkle paprika on top and serve as a Paleo snack.

Nutrition: calories 228, fat 22,1, fiber 3,1, carbs 7,9, protein 3,2

Chapter 6 -   Meat Recipes

45) Cilantro Beef Mix

Preparation Time: 10 minutes   **Cooking Time: 35 minutes**   Servings:4

Ingredients:

- 1 pound beef, ground
- 1 teaspoon cumin seeds, toasted
- 1 pound sweet potatoes, cubed
- 3 tablespoons ghee
- 2 onions, chopped
- 1 small ginger pieces, grated

- 1 Serrano pepper, chopped
- 2 teaspoons coriander powder
- 2 teaspoons garam masala
- Black pepper to the taste
- 1 cup steamed broccoli
- A handful cilantro, chopped

Directions:

⇒ Heat up a pan with 2 tablespoons ghee over medium heat, add sweet potato cubes, stir, cook them for 20 minutes and transfer them to a bowl.

⇒ Heat up the same pan over medium heat, add cumin, Serrano pepper and onion, stir and cook for 4 minutes.

⇒ Add beef, ginger, coriander, garam masala, cayenne and black pepper, stir and cook for 5 minutes more.

⇒ Add broccoli and sweet potatoes, stir, cook for 5 minutes more, divide between plates and serve with cilantro on top.

Nutrition: calories 465, fat 17,1, fiber 6,8, carbs 39,4, protein 37,8

46) Beef Stir Fry

Preparation Time: 10 minutes   **Cooking Time: 15 minutes**   Servings:4

Ingredients:

- 1 yellow onion, chopped
- 1 pound beef, ground
- 1 napa cabbage head, shredded
- 1 carrot, grated

- A pinch of sea salt
- Black pepper to taste
- 2 tablespoons coconut oil, melted

Directions:

⇒ Heat up a pan with the oil over medium-high heat, add the onion and beef, stir and brown them for 5 minutes.

⇒ Add carrots, cabbage, a pinch of salt and black pepper to taste, stir and cook for 10 minutes more.

⇒ Divide between plates and serve.

Nutrition: calories 314, fat 14,3, fiber 3,1, carbs 8,7, protein 38

47) Ground Beef and Veggies

Preparation Time: 10 minutes   **Cooking Time: 12 minutes**   Servings:4

Ingredients:

- 1 pound beef, ground
- 1 apple, cored, peeled and chopped
- 1 yellow onion, chopped
- 3 cups Brussels sprouts, shredded

- A pinch of sea salt
- Black pepper to taste
- 3 tablespoons ghee, melted

Directions:

⇒ Heat up a pan with the ghee over medium-high heat, add the beef, stir and brown for 2 minutes.

⇒ Add Brussels sprouts, stir and cook for 3 minutes more.

⇒ Add onion and the apple, stir and cook for 5 minutes more.

⇒ Add a pinch of sea salt and black pepper, stir, cook for 1 minute more, divide between plates and serve.

Nutrition: calories 363, fat 17, fiber 4,4, carbs 16,3, protein 27,1

48) Beef and Olives Mix

Preparation Time: 10 minutes **Cooking Time: 12 minutes** **Servings:2**

Ingredients:

- 1 big oyster mushroom, chopped
- 2 tablespoons almonds, chopped
- 2 tablespoons ghee, melted
- 4 ounces beef, ground
- ½ teaspoon chili flakes
- A pinch of sea salt
- White pepper to taste
- 1 tablespoon capers, chopped
- ¼ cup kalamata olives, pitted
- 1 tablespoon coconut butter
- 3 ounces spinach leaves, torn

Directions:

⇒ Heat up a pan with the ghee over medium-high heat, add mushroom, stir and cook for 3 minutes.

⇒ Add almonds, beef, chili flakes, a pinch of salt and white pepper, stir and cook for 7 minutes.

⇒ Add the coconut butter, capers, olives and spinach, stir, cook for a couple more minutes, divide into 2 bowls and serve.

Nutrition: calories 484, fat 22,6, fiber 5,9, carbs 21,7, protein 49,5

49) Beef and Carrots Mix

Preparation Time: 10 minutes **Cooking Time: 16 minutes** **Servings:4**

Ingredients:

- 6 garlic cloves, minced
- 2 red chilies, chopped
- 1 tablespoon coconut oil, melted
- 1 yellow onion, chopped
- 1 and ½ pounds beef, ground
- A pinch of sea salt and black pepper
- 3 cups basil, chopped
- ½ cup chicken stock
- 2 cups carrot, grated
- 4 tablespoons lime juice
- 2 tablespoons coconut aminos
- 1 tablespoon olive oil

Directions:

⇒ Heat up a pan with the oil over medium heat, add the onions and a pinch of salt, stir and cook for 4 minutes.

⇒ Add garlic and chili peppers, stir and cook for 1 minute more.

⇒ Add beef and black pepper, stir and brown everything for 8 minutes.

⇒ Add stock and half of the basil, stir and cook for 2 minutes more.

⇒ In a bowl, mix carrots with 1 tablespoon lime juice, the rest of the basil and the olive oil and stir well.

⇒ In another bowl, mix coconut aminos with the rest of the lime juice and whisk well.

⇒ Divide the beef mix and carrots into bowls, drizzle the coconut aminos mix on top and serve.

Nutrition: calories 439, fat 20,1, fiber 2,4, carbs 11,6, protein 51,4

50) Beef with Squash and Peppers

Preparation Time: 10 minutes **Cooking Time: 30 minutes** **Servings:4**

Ingredients:

- 1 pound beef, ground
- 1 tablespoon parsley flakes
- 2 big tomatoes, chopped
- 2 yellow squash, chopped
- 2 green bell peppers, chopped
- 1 yellow onion, chopped
- A pinch of sea salt
- Black pepper to taste

Directions:

⇒ Heat up a pan over medium-high heat, add onion and beef, stir and cook for 10 minutes.

⇒ Add tomatoes, stir and cook for a 2 more minutes.

⇒ Add parsley flakes, black pepper and a pinch of sea salt, stir and cook for 10 minutes more.

⇒ Add bell pepper pieces and squash ones, stir, cook for 10 minutes, divide between plates and serve.

Nutrition: calories 273, fat 7,6, fiber 3,6, carbs 14, protein 37,3

51) Savory Beef Salad

Preparation Time: 10 minutes   **Cooking Time: 25 minutes**   **Servings:4**

Ingredients:

- 1 pound beef, ground
- 1 tablespoon olive oil
- 2 garlic cloves, minced
- 1 yellow onion, chopped
- A pinch of sea salt
- Black pepper to taste
- 1 tablespoon savory, dried

- 1 tablespoon parsley, dried
- 2 tablespoons oregano, dried
- 3 ounces kale, chopped
- 3 ounces endives, chopped
- ¼ cup kalamata olives, pitted and sliced
- ¼ cup green olives, pitted and sliced

Directions:

⇒ Heat up a pan with the oil over medium-high heat, add garlic, onion, a pinch of salt and black pepper, stir and cook for 3 minutes.

⇒ Add beef, stir and cook for 10 minutes.

⇒ Add endives, kale, savory, oregano and parsley, stir and cook for 5 minutes more.

⇒ Add green and kalamata olives, stir, place in preheated broiler and broil for 4 minutes over medium heat.

⇒ Divide into bowls and serve.

Nutrition: calories 318, fat 14,4, fiber 4,3, carbs 10,9, protein 36,5

52) Coconut Beef

Preparation Time: 10 minutes   **Cooking Time: 35 minutes**   **Servings:4**

Ingredients:

- 1 teaspoon mustard seeds
- 2 tablespoons olive oil
- 1 Serrano pepper, chopped
- 1 yellow onion, chopped
- 1 tablespoon garlic, minced
- ¼ cup water
- 2 teaspoons garam masala
- ¼ teaspoon chili powder

- ½ teaspoon turmeric powder
- 1 teaspoon coriander powder
- 1 pound beef, ground
- A pinch of sea salt
- Black pepper to taste
- 3 carrot, chopped
- 10 ounces coconut milk

Directions:

⇒ Heat up a pan with the oil over medium-high heat, add mustard seeds, stir and toast them for 1 minute.

⇒ Add Serrano pepper and the onion, stir and cook for 5 minutes.

⇒ Add the garlic, stir and cook for 1 minute.

⇒ Add beef, salt, black pepper, coriander powder, turmeric, chili and garam masala, stir and cook for 10 minutes.

⇒ Add carrot and the water, stir and cook for 5 minutes more.

⇒ Add coconut milk, stir well and cook for 15 minutes.

⇒ Divide curry into bowls and serve.

Nutrition: calories 472, fat 31,3, fiber 3,6, carbs 12,4, protein 37,1

53) Thai Ground Beef

Preparation Time: 10 minutes   **Cooking Time: 30 minutes**   **Servings:4**

Ingredients:

- 1 yellow onion, chopped
- 3 Thai chilies, chopped
- 2 tablespoons avocado oil
- 1 pound beef, ground
- 1-inch ginger piece, grated
- 3 garlic cloves, minced
- ½ teaspoon cumin
- ½ teaspoon turmeric powder
- A pinch of sea salt
- Black pepper to taste
- 1 tablespoon red curry paste
- 1 cup tomato sauce
- 1 broccoli head, florets separated
- 1 handful basil, chopped
- 2 teaspoons lime juice
- 2 tablespoons coconut aminos

Directions:

⇒ Heat up a pan with the oil over medium heat, add chilies and onion, stir and cook for 5 minutes.

⇒ Add salt, ginger, garlic, cumin, turmeric, black pepper, cayenne and beef, stir and cook for 10 minutes.

⇒ Add broccoli and curry paste, stir and cook for 1 minute more.

⇒ Add basil, tomato paste and coconut aminos, stir, bring to a simmer, cover, reduce heat to medium-low and cook for 15 minutes.

⇒ Add lime juice, stir, divide into bowls and serve.

Nutrition: calories 163, fat 3,7, fiber 5,7, carbs 28,6, protein 5,4

54) Beef and Lettuce Mix

Preparation Time: 10 minutes   **Cooking Time: 8 minutes**   **Servings:4**

Ingredients:

- 2 garlic cloves, minced
- 1 sweet onion, chopped
- 1 tablespoon coconut oil, melted
- 1 pound beef, ground
- 1 cup cherry tomatoes, chopped
- 1 dill pickle, chopped
- 1 lettuce head, leaves separated and torn
- A pinch of sea salt and black pepper

  For the dressing:
- 2 tablespoons water
- 4 tablespoons mayonnaise
- 1 tablespoon yellow onion, chopped
- 1 teaspoon balsamic vinegar

Directions:

⇒ Heat up a pan with the oil over medium heat, add garlic and onion, stir and cook for 2 minutes.

⇒ Add beef, salt and black pepper, stir, cook for 8 minutes more and take off heat.

⇒ In a salad bowl, combine beef mix and with lettuce, the pickle and cherry tomatoes.

⇒ In another bowl, mix water with the mayo, yellow onion and the vinegar and whisk well.

⇒ Drizzle this over salad, toss to coat and serve.

Nutrition: calories 332, fat 15,7, fiber 1,9, carbs 11,1, protein 35,8

55) Veal and Zucchini Wraps

Preparation Time: 10 minutes   **Cooking Time: 20 minutes**   **Servings:4**

Ingredients:

- 2 zucchinis, cut into quarters
- 8 veal scallops
- 2 tablespoons olive oil
- 2 teaspoons garlic powder
- ¼ cup balsamic vinegar
- A pinch of sea salt
- Black pepper to taste

Directions:

⇒ Flatten veal scallops with a meat tenderizer and season them with salt and black pepper.

⇒ Season zucchini salt, black pepper and garlic powder, place on preheated grill over medium-high heat, cook for 2 minutes on each side and transfer to a working surface.

⇒ Roll veal around each zucchini piece.

⇒ In a bowl, mix oil with balsamic vinegar and whisk well.

⇒ Brush veal rolls with this mix, place them on your grill and cook for 3 minutes on each side.

⇒ Serve right away.

Nutrition: calories 136, fat 7,7, fiber 1,2, carbs 5,9, protein 11,5

56) Beef and Mushrooms

Preparation Time: 10 minutes   **Cooking Time: 3 hours**   **Servings:4**

Ingredients:

- 1 yellow onion, sliced
- 3 garlic cloves, minced
- 1 cup beef stock
- 2 tablespoons coconut oil, melted
- 3 pounds beef, cubed
- A pinch of sea salt and black pepper
- 8 ounces carrots, sliced
- 8 ounces mushrooms, sliced
- 1 teaspoon thyme, chopped

Directions:

⇒ Heat up a Dutch oven with half of the oil over medium-high heat, add beef cubes, season with salt and black pepper, brown for 2 minutes on each side and transfer to a bowl.

⇒ Heat up the same Dutch oven over medium heat, add garlic, stir and cook for 2 minutes.

⇒ Add stock, stir well and heat it up.

⇒ Return meat to the pot, stir, place in the oven at 250 degrees F and roast for 3 hours.

⇒ In a bowl, mix carrots with mushrooms, the rest of the oil, salt, black pepper and thyme, stir well, spread these into a pan, place in the oven at 250 degrees F and roast them for 15 minutes.

⇒ Divide beef and juices between plates and serve with roasted veggies on the side.

Nutrition: calories 745, fat 28,4, fiber 2,7, carbs 10,9, protein 106,6

57) Thyme Steaks Mix

Preparation Time: 10 minutes   **Cooking Time: 20 minutes**   **Servings:4**

Ingredients:

- 1 cup beef stock
- 2 tablespoons shallots, chopped
- 2 garlic cloves, minced
- 1 cup blueberries
- 4 medium flank steaks
- 2 tablespoons ghee, melted
- 1 teaspoon thyme, chopped
- A pinch of sea salt
- Black pepper to taste

Directions:

⇒ Heat up a pan with the ghee over medium heat, add shallot and garlic, stir and cook for 4 minutes.

⇒ Add thyme, stock, a pinch of salt and black pepper, stir, bring to a simmer and cook for 10 minutes.

⇒ Add blueberries, stir and cook for 2 minutes more

⇒ Put the steaks on preheated grill over medium-high heat, cook for 4 minutes son each side and transfer to plates.

⇒ Drizzle the blueberry sauce on top and serve.

Nutrition: calories 708, fat 33,3, fiber 1, carbs 6,8, protein 90,3

58) Garlic Beef and Greens

Preparation Time: 10 minutes   **Cooking Time: 20 minutes**   **Servings:4**

Ingredients:

- 1 onion, sliced
- 12 baby bok choy heads, halved
- 2 pound beef sirloin, cut into strips
- 2 garlic cloves, minced
- 3 tablespoons coconut oil

- 5 red chilies, dried and chopped
- A pinch of sea salt
- Black pepper to taste
- 1 teaspoon ginger, grated

Directions:

⇒ Heat up a pan with the oil over high heat, add chilies, garlic and ginger, stir and cook for 1 minute.

⇒ Add beef, stir, cook for 3 minutes and transfer to a bowl.

⇒ Heat up the pan again over medium-high heat, add onion, stir and cook for 2 minutes.

⇒ Add bok choy, stir and cook for 4 minutes more.

⇒ Return beef mix to the pan, stir, cook for 1 minute more, divide between plates and serve hot.

Nutrition: calories 854, fat 29,5, fiber 26,1, carbs 58,8, protein 107,1

59) Parsley Lamb Mix

Preparation Time: 10 minutes   **Cooking Time: 7 minutes**   **Servings:4**

Ingredients:

- 8 lamb chops
- 2 tablespoons ras el hanout
- 1 teaspoon olive oil
- For the sauce:
- ¼ cup parsley, chopped
- 2 tablespoons mint, chopped
- 3 garlic cloves, minced

- 2 tablespoons lemon zest
- ¼ cup olive oil
- ½ teaspoon smoked paprika
- 1 teaspoon red pepper flakes
- 2 tablespoons lemon juice
- A pinch of sea salt
- Black pepper to taste

Directions:

⇒ Rub lamb chops with ras el hanout and 1 teaspoon oil, put them on preheated grill over medium-high heat, cook for 2 minutes on each side and divide them between plates.

⇒ In a food processor, mix parsley with mint, garlic, lemon zest, ¼ cup oil, paprika, pepper flakes, lemon juice, a pinch of salt and black pepper and pulse really well.

⇒ Drizzle this over lamb chops and serve.

Nutrition: calories 551, fat 32,6, fiber 0,8, carbs 2,4, protein 60,2

60) Broiled Lamb

Preparation Time: 10 minutes   **Cooking Time: 10 minutes**   **Servings:4**

Ingredients:

- 4 lamb chops
- 12 rosemary springs
- 4 garlic cloves, halved

- ½ teaspoon black peppercorns
- 3 tablespoons avocado oil
- A pinch of sea salt

Directions:

⇒ In a bowl, mix lamb chops with salt, black peppercorns and oil, rub well, place the chops in a lined baking sheet and add the garlic halves on top.

⇒ Rub rosemary into your palms and add over lamb chops.

⇒ Introduce everything in preheated broiler over medium-high heat for 10 minutes, divide between plates and serve.

Nutrition: calories 634, fat 25,6, fiber 1,3, carbs 2,8, protein 92,3

61) Grilled Lamb Mix

Preparation Time: 2 hours   **Cooking Time: 10 minutes**   Servings:4

Ingredients:

- 4 lamb chops
- 2 garlic cloves, minced
- 1 tablespoon lavender, chopped
- 2 tablespoons rosemary, chopped

- A pinch of sea salt
- Black pepper to taste
- 1 tablespoon ghee
- 3 small orange peel, grated

Directions:

⇒ In a bowl, mix lamb chops with garlic, lavender, rosemary, orange peel, a pinch of salt and black pepper, rub well and keep in the fridge for 2 hours.

⇒ Heat up your grill over medium-high heat, grease with the ghee, place lamb chops on it, grill for 5 minutes on each side, divide between plates and serve with a side salad on the side.

Nutrition: calories 645, fat 27,4, fiber 0,7, carbs 1,8, protein 92

62) Lamb Chops and Eggplant Mix

Preparation Time: 15 minutes   **Cooking Time: 3 hours and 10 minutes**   Servings:4

Ingredients:

- 4 lamb chops
- 1 tablespoon ghee, melted
- A pinch of sea salt and black pepper
- 1 cup yellow onion, chopped
- 7 ounces tomato paste
- 2 garlic cloves, minced
- 3 cups water

- 8 ounces white mushrooms, halved
- For the eggplant puree:
- Juice of 1 lemon
- ¼ teaspoon white pepper
- 2 eggplants
- 4 tablespoons ghee
- A pinch of sea salt

Directions:

⇒ Place eggplants on your preheated grill, cook for 30 minutes, flipping them from time to time, leave them to cool down and peel.

⇒ In a food processor, mix eggplant flesh with salt, white pepper, lemon juice and 4 tablespoons ghee and pulse really well.

⇒ Heat up a pot with 1 tablespoon ghee, add lamb chops, season with salt and black pepper to taste, stir, brown them for a 3 minutes on each side and transfer to a plate.

⇒ Heat up the pot again over medium-high heat, add the onion, stir and cook for 2 minutes.

⇒ Add garlic, stir and cook for 1 minute more.

⇒ Add mushrooms and tomato paste, stir and cook for 3 minutes more.

⇒ Add water, return lamb chops to the pan as well, stir, bring to a simmer, cover pot, reduce heat to medium-low heat and cook everything for 2 hours and 20 minutes.

⇒ Divide lamb chops between plates and serve with the eggplant puree on the side.

Nutrition: calories 895, fat 41,1, fiber 13, carbs 31,7, protein 98,9

Chapter 7 -   Seafood & Fish Recipes

63) Shrimp and Garlic Sauce

Preparation Time: 10 minutes   **Cooking Time: 8 minutes**   Servings:4

Ingredients:

- 1 pound shrimp, deveined
- 2 tablespoons parsley, minced
- 2 garlic cloves, minced
- 3 tablespoons lemon juice
- 2 tablespoons olive oil
- A pinch of sea salt
- Black pepper to taste

Directions:

⇒ Heat up a pan with the oil over medium heat, add the shrimp, and cook for 3 minutes on each side.

⇒ Add garlic, parsley, lemon juice, salt and pepper, toss, cook for 2 more minutes, divide into bowls and serve.

Nutrition: calories 200, fat 9, fiber 0,1, carbs 2,6, protein 26,1

64) Shrimp Salad

Preparation Time: 10 minutes   **Cooking Time: 6 minutes**   Servings:2

Ingredients:

- 2 cucumbers, cut with a spiralizer
- 1 pound shrimp, peeled and deveined
- 4 garlic cloves, minced
- 2 tablespoons olive oil
- 2 tablespoons lemon juice
- 2 tablespoons chives, minced
- A pinch of sea salt
- Black pepper to taste

Directions:

⇒ Heat up a pan with the oil over medium heat, add garlic, stir and cook for 3 minutes.

⇒ Add the shrimp and the lemon juice, stir, cook for 4 minutes more and transfer to a bowl.

⇒ Add cucumber noodles, salt, pepper and the chives, toss and serve.

Nutrition: calories 448, fat 18,3, fiber 1,8, carbs 16,8, protein 54,2

65) Dill Salmon

Preparation Time: 10 minutes   **Cooking Time: 20 minutes**   Servings:4

Ingredients:

- 1 cup walnuts, chopped
- 4 salmon fillets, boneless
- ¼ cup lemon juice
- 2 tablespoons stevia
- 1 teaspoon dill, chopped
- A pinch of sea salt
- Black pepper to taste
- 1 tablespoon mustard

Directions:

⇒ In a bowl, mix the walnuts with mustard, stevia, lemon juice, a pinch of salt, black pepper and dill and stir well.

⇒ Spread this over salmon fillets, press well, place them on a lined baking sheet, place in the oven at 375 degrees F and bake for 20 minutes.

⇒ Divide salmon between plates and serve with a side salad.

Nutrition: calories 446, fat 30,4, fiber 2,6, carbs 4,5, protein 42,9

66) Calamari and Kale Mix

Preparation Time: 15 minutes   **Cooking Time: 50 minutes**   **Servings:4**

Ingredients:

- 4 big calamari, tentacles separated and chopped
- 2 tablespoons parsley, chopped
- 5 ounces kale, chopped
- 2 garlic cloves, minced
- 1 red bell pepper, chopped
- 1 teaspoon oregano, dried
- 15 ounces homemade tomato puree
- Olive oil
- 1 yellow onion, chopped
- A pinch of sea salt
- Black pepper to taste

Directions:

⇒ Heat up a pan with some olive oil over medium heat, add onion and garlic, stir and cook for 2 minutes.

⇒ Add bell pepper, stir and cook for 3 minutes.

⇒ Add calamari tentacles, stir and cook for 6 minutes more.

⇒ Add kale, a pinch of sea salt and black pepper, stir, cook for a couple more minutes and take off heat.

⇒ Stuff calamari tubes with this mix and secure with toothpicks.

⇒ Heat up a pan with some olive oil over medium-high heat, add calamari, brown them for 2 minutes on each side and then mix with tomato puree.

⇒ Also add parsley, oregano and some black pepper to the pan, stir gently, cover, reduce heat to medium-low and simmer for 40 minutes.

⇒ Divide stuffed calamari on plates and serve.

Nutrition: calories 637, fat 23,7, fiber 6,3, carbs 57,9, protein 42,9

67) Maple Salmon

Preparation Time: 10 minutes   **Cooking Time: 12 minutes**   **Servings:4**

Ingredients:

- 2 tablespoons dill, chopped
- 4 salmon fillets, boneless
- 2 tablespoons chives, chopped
- 1/3 cup maple syrup
- A drizzle of olive oil
- 3 tablespoons balsamic vinegar
- A pinch of sea salt
- Black pepper to taste
- Lime wedges for serving

Directions:

⇒ Heat up a pan with the oil over medium-high heat, add fish fillets, season them with a pinch of sea salt and black pepper, cook for 3 minutes, cover pan and cook for 6 minutes more.

⇒ Add balsamic vinegar and maple syrup and cook for 3 minutes basting fish with this mix.

⇒ Add dill and chives, cook for 1 minute, divide the fish between plates and serve with lime wedges on the side.

Nutrition: calories 346, fat 14,7, fiber 0,7, carbs 20,4, protein 35

68) Mustard Cod

Preparation Time: 10 minutes   **Cooking Time: 20 minutes**   **Servings:4**

Ingredients:

- 1 tablespoon cilantro, chopped
- 4 medium cod fillets, boneless
- ¼ cup ghee
- 2 garlic cloves, minced
- 2 tablespoons olive oil
- 2 tablespoons lemon juice

- 3 tablespoons prosciutto, chopped
- 1 teaspoon Dijon mustard
- 1 shallot, chopped
- A pinch of sea salt
- Black pepper to taste

Directions:

⇒ In a bowl, mix mustard with ghee, garlic, cilantro, shallot, lemon juice, prosciutto, salt and pepper and whisk well.

⇒ Heat up a pan with the oil over medium-high heat, add the fish fillets, season them with some black pepper and cook for 4 minutes on each side.

⇒ Spread mustard and ghee mix over fish, transfer everything to a lined baking sheet, place in the oven at 425 degrees F and bake for 10 minutes.

⇒ Divide fish between plates and serve.

Nutrition: calories 279, fat 21,2, fiber 0,1, carbs 1,3, protein 21,7

69) Halibut and Peppers Slaw

Preparation Time: 15 minutes   **Cooking Time: 10 minutes**   **Servings:4**

Ingredients:

- 4 medium halibut fillets, skinless, boneless
- 2 teaspoons olive oil
- 4 teaspoons lemon juice
- 1 garlic clove, minced
- 1 teaspoon sweet paprika
- A pinch of sea salt
- Black pepper to taste

For the salsa:

- ¼ cup green onions, chopped
- 1 cup red bell pepper, chopped
- 4 teaspoons oregano, chopped
- 1 small habanero pepper, chopped
- 1 garlic clove, minced
- ¼ cup lemon juice

Directions:

⇒ In a bowl, mix red bell pepper with habanero, green onion, ¼ cup lemon juice, 1 garlic clove, oregano, a pinch of sea salt and black pepper, stir well and keep in the fridge for now.

⇒ In a large bowl, mix paprika, olive oil, 1 garlic clove and 4 teaspoons lemon juice and stir well.

⇒ Add fish, rub well, cover bowl and leave aside for 10 minutes.

⇒ Place marinated fish under preheated broiler over medium-high heat, season with a pinch of sea salt and black pepper, cook for 4 minutes on each side and divide between plates.

⇒ Top fish with the salsa you've made earlier and serve.

Nutrition: calories 402, fat 8,7, fiber 0,2, carbs 0,6, protein 75,7

70) Salmon Rolls

Preparation Time: 10 minutes   **Cooking Time: 20 minutes**   **Servings:4**

Ingredients:

- 6 cabbage leaves, sliced in half
- 4 medium salmon steaks, skinless
- 2 red bell peppers, chopped
- Some coconut oil

- 1 yellow onion, chopped
- A pinch of sea salt
- Black pepper to taste

Directions:

⇒ Put water in a large saucepan, bring to a boil over medium-high heat, add cabbage leaves, blanch them for 2 minutes, transfer to a bowl filled with cold water and pat dry.

⇒ Season salmon steaks with a pinch of sea salt and black pepper to taste and wrap each in 3 cabbage leaf halves.

⇒ Heat up a pan with some coconut oil over medium-high heat, add onion and bell pepper, stir and cook for 4 minutes.

⇒ Add wrapped salmon, place pan in the oven at 350 degrees F and bake for 12 minutes.

⇒ Divide salmon and veggies between plates and serve.

Nutrition: calories 271, fat 11,2, fiber 2, carbs 8,4, protein 35,7

71) Cod and Coconut Sauce

Preparation Time: 10 minutes   **Cooking Time: 15 minutes**   **Servings:4**

Ingredients:

- 1 tablespoon chives, chopped
- 4 medium cod fillets
- 1 tablespoon thyme, chopped
- 1 tablespoon parsley, chopped
- Grated zest of ½ lemon
- 1 shallot, chopped

- ¾ cup coconut milk
- 6 tablespoons ghee
- 2 garlic cloves
- A pinch of sea salt
- Black pepper to taste

Directions:

⇒ In a bowl, mix garlic with ghee, shallots, chives, parsley and thyme and stir well.

⇒ Season cod with a pinch of salt and black pepper to taste.

⇒ Heat up a pan over medium heat, add herbed sauce and the fish, toss to coat and cook for 2 minutes on each side.

⇒ Transfer fish to a lined baking sheet, place in the oven at 400 degrees F and bake for 7 minutes.

⇒ Heat up the pan with the herbed sauce over medium heat, add lemon zest and coconut milk, stir and bring to a simmer over medium heat.

⇒ Divide fish between plates, drizzle the herbed sauce on top and serve.

Nutrition: calories 372, fat 31, fiber 1,7, carbs 5,3, protein 21,5

72) Pesto Salmon Mix

Preparation Time: 10 minutes   **Cooking Time: 15 minutes**   **Servings:4**

Ingredients:

- 4 salmon fillets, skin on
- 1 tablespoon red bell pepper, chopped
- 1 shallot, chopped
- 2 tablespoon basil, chopped
- ½ cup cherry tomatoes, cut in quarters

- 2 garlic cloves, minced
- ½ cup sun-dried tomatoes, chopped
- 3 tablespoons olive oil
- A pinch of sea salt
- Black pepper to taste

Directions:

⇒ In a food processor, mix sun-dried tomatoes with garlic, oil, basil, shallots, a pinch of sea salt and black pepper and blend well.

⇒ Rub salmon with some of this mix, place under preheated broiler over medium-high heat, cook for 12 minutes flipping once and divide between plates.

⇒ Add the rest of the tomato pesto on top and serve with cherry tomatoes and bell pepper pieces on the side.

Nutrition: calories 343, fat 21,6, fiber 0,7, carbs 4,1, protein 35,2

Chapter 8 -   Salad Recipes

73) Beet and Walnuts Salad

Preparation Time: 10 minutes   **Cooking Time: 0 minutes**   **Servings:2**

Ingredients:

- 2 beetroots, cooked, peeled and cut into medium pieces
- 1/3 cup walnuts, chopped
- ¼ teaspoon cinnamon powder
- ½ teaspoon maple syrup
- 2 tablespoons olive oil

- 1 tablespoon vinegar
- ½ teaspoon mustard
- 3 cups salad leaves, torn
- A pinch of sea salt
- Black pepper to taste

Directions:

⇒ In a salad bowl, combine all the ingredients, toss and serve.

Nutrition: calories 336, fat 26,9, fiber 3,5, carbs 20,2, protein 9,5

74) Turkey and Arugula Salad

Preparation Time: 10 minutes   **Cooking Time: 20 minutes**   **Servings:4**

Ingredients:

- 4 cups arugula
- 1 tablespoon rosemary, chopped
- 2 green onions, chopped
- 10 ounce turkey meat, sliced
- 1 tablespoon olive oil
- 2 garlic cloves, minced
- 4 sweet potatoes, peeled and cubed

- A pinch of sea salt
- Black pepper to taste

  For the salad dressing:
- 2 teaspoons mustard
- 2 tablespoons apple vinegar
- 4 tablespoons olive oil
- ½ teaspoon lemon juice

Directions:

⇒ Heat up a pan with the olive oil over medium heat, add sweet potatoes, stir and cook for 7 minutes.

⇒ Add a pinch of salt, black pepper, rosemary and garlic, stir and cook for 6 minutes more.

⇒ Add turkey meat slices, stir, cook for 3 minutes, take off heat, cool down and transfer everything to a salad bowl.

⇒ Add green onions and arugula and stir.

⇒ In a small bowl, mix olive oil with lemon juice, vinegar, mustard and some black pepper and whisk well.

⇒ Add this to salad, toss to coat and serve.

Nutrition: calories 468, fat 22,1, fiber 7,3, carbs 44,7, protein 24,3

75) Mint Shrimp and Fennel Salad

Preparation Time: 10 minutes   **Cooking Time: 4 minutes**   **Servings:4**

Ingredients:

- 2 pounds shrimp, deveined
- A pinch of sea salt
- Black pepper to taste
- 2 tablespoons olive oil
- 4 ounces watermelon radish, thinly sliced
- 4 ounces radishes, sliced

- ½ cup fennel bulb, chopped
- 4 green onions, chopped
- 1 teaspoon maple syrup
- 2 tablespoons lemon juice
- ¼ cup mint, chopped
- 2 tablespoons paleo mayonnaise

Directions:

⇒ Heat up a pan with the oil over medium-high heat, add shrimp, season with a pinch of salt and some black pepper, cook for 2 minutes on each side and transfer them to a salad bowl.

⇒ Add watermelon radish, radishes, fennel and onions and stir gently.

⇒ In a small bowl, mix maple syrup with lemon juice, mint and mayo and whisk well.

⇒ Add this to salad, toss to coat well and serve.

Nutrition: calories 411, fat 15,1, fiber 2,2, carbs 13,8, protein 53,3

76) Steak and Peppers Salad

Preparation Time: 10 minutes   **Cooking Time: 0 minutes**   **Servings:4**

Ingredients:

- 6 cups romaine lettuce, chopped
- 1 red onion, chopped
- 1 yellow bell pepper, chopped
- 1 red bell pepper, chopped
- A pinch of sea salt
- Black pepper to taste

- 1 cucumber, sliced
- ½ cup kalamata olives, pitted and sliced
- ¼ cup parsley, chopped
- ¾ pound flank steak, cooked and sliced
- 1 tablespoon olive oil

Directions:

⇒ In a salad bowl, mix lettuce with onion, yellow bell pepper, red bell pepper, cucumber, olives, parsley and steak slices and toss well.

⇒ Add a pinch of salt, black pepper and the oil, toss to coat well and serve.

Nutrition: calories 259, fat 12,7, fiber 2,6, carbs 11,3, protein 25,4

77) Beet and Parsley Salad

Preparation Time: 10 minutes   **Cooking Time: 0 minutes**   **Servings:4**

Ingredients:

- ½ cup walnuts, chopped
- ¼ cup Paleo mayo anise
- 1 and ½ pounds beets, roasted, peeled and grated
- ½ cup raisins

- 2 garlic cloves, minced
- ¼ cup parsley, chopped
- A pinch of sea salt
- Black pepper to taste

Directions:

⇒ In a salad bowl, mix grated beets with walnuts, raisins, garlic, parsley, salt and pepper and stir.

⇒ Add mayo, stir well and serve cold.

Nutrition: calories 321, fat 19,7, fiber 3, carbs 3, protein 8

78) Cucumber Salad

Preparation Time: 10 minutes   **Cooking Time: 0 minutes**   **Servings:4**

Ingredients:

- 2 tablespoons balsamic vinegar
- 3 tablespoons olive oil
- 1 teaspoon oregano, chopped
- 1 and ½ pounds cucumber, sliced
- 1 cup mixed colored tomatoes, halved
- 2 tablespoons mint, chopped

- ½ cup red onion, chopped
- 2 tablespoons parsley, chopped
- 2 tablespoons dill, chopped
- A pinch of sea salt
- Black pepper to taste

Directions:

⇒ In a bowl, mix cucumber with tomatoes, onion, mint, parsley, oregano, dill, salt and pepper and stir.

⇒ Add vinegar and oil, toss to coat and serve.

Nutrition: calories 136, fat 10,9, fiber 2,3, carbs 10.2, protein 2,1

79) Chard and Walnuts Salad

Preparation Time: 10 minutes   **Cooking Time: 3 minutes**   **Servings:4**

Ingredients:

- 1 garlic clove, minced
- 1 shallot, chopped
- 1 tablespoon rosemary, chopped
- A pinch of sea salt
- Black pepper to taste

- 2 tablespoons avocado oil
- 1 bunch Swiss chard, sliced
- 1 and ½ cup walnuts, halved
- 1 tablespoon vinegar
- 1 tablespoon lemon juice

Directions:

⇒ Heat up a pan with the oil over medium-high heat, add garlic, rosemary, shallot, a pinch of salt and black pepper, stir and cook for 3 minutes.

⇒ Add walnuts, stir, reduce heat and cook for a few seconds more.

⇒ In a salad bowl, mix Swiss chard with vinegar, lemon juice and shallots mix and toss to coat.

Nutrition: calories 218, fat 20,6, fiber 2,9, carbs 7, protein 5,1

80) Balsamic Cabbage Salad

Preparation Time: 10 minutes   **Cooking Time: 6 minutes**   **Servings:4**

Ingredients:

- 1 red cabbage head, shredded
- 2 tablespoons olive oil
- A pinch of sea salt
- Black pepper to taste
- ¼ cup balsamic vinegar

- ½ teaspoon oregano, dried
- 1 yellow onion, chopped
- 1 tablespoon maple syrup
- 2 figs, cut into quarters
- A handful oregano, chopped

Directions:

⇒ In a bowl mix cabbage with a pinch of salt and some black pepper, stir well and leave aside.

⇒ Heat up a pan with half of the oil over medium heat, add onion, stir and cook for 4 minutes.

⇒ Add dried oregano and vinegar, stir, cook for 5 minutes and take off heat.

⇒ Add maple syrup, some black pepper and stir well.

⇒ In a salad bowl, mix squeezed cabbage with onions mix, figs and the rest of the oil, toss to coat and serve with fresh oregano on top.

Nutrition: calories 156, fat 7,3, fiber 6,1, carbs 23,4, protein 2,9

81) Shrimp and Turkey Salad

Preparation Time: 10 minutes   **Cooking Time: 4 minutes**   **Servings:4**

Ingredients:

- 5 oz turkey meat, cooked and chopped
- 1 tablespoon olive oil
- 1 pound shrimp, peeled and deveined
- 1 teaspoon garlic powder
- A pinch of sea salt
- Black pepper to taste
- 6 cups romaine lettuce leaves, chopped
- 4 eggs, hard-boiled, peeled and chopped

- 1-pint cherry tomatoes, halved
- 1 avocado, pitted, peeled and chopped
- For the vinaigrette:
- 1 garlic clove, minced
- 2 tablespoons Paleo mayonnaise
- 2 tablespoon vinegar
- 3 tablespoons avocado oil

Directions:

⇒ In a bowl mix garlic with mayo, vinegar and avocado oil, whisk well and leave aside for now.

⇒ Heat up a pan with the olive oil over medium-high heat, add shrimp, season with a pinch of salt, some black pepper and garlic powder, cook for 2 minutes, flip, cook for 2 minutes more and transfer them to a salad bowl.

⇒ Add tomatoes, avocado pieces, lettuce leaves, turkey and egg pieces and stir.

⇒ Add the vinaigrette you've made earlier, toss to coat and serve.

Nutrition: calories 561, fat 37,2, fiber 5,1, carbs13,2, protein 44

82) Tomato, Greens and Shrimp Salad

Preparation Time: 1 hour   **Cooking Time: 8 minutes**   **Servings:4**

Ingredients:

- ¼ cup ghee, melted
- ½ teaspoon dill, dried
- ¼ teaspoon smoked paprika
- A pinch of sea salt
- Black pepper to taste
- 2 small shallots, already cooked and chopped

- 12 ounces shrimp, peeled and deveined
- 4 cups mixed salad greens
- 1 avocado, pitted, peeled and chopped
- A handful cherry tomatoes, halved
- 2 tablespoons scallions, chopped

Directions:

⇒ In a bowl, mix ghee with a pinch of salt, black pepper, dill and paprika and stir well.

⇒ Put shrimp in a bowl, add half of the ghee mix over them, toss well and leave aside in the fridge for 1 hour.

⇒ Heat up a pan over medium-high heat, add shrimp, cook for 3 minutes on each side and transfer to a bowl.

⇒ Add the rest of the ghee mix, shallots, mixed greens, avocado, tomatoes and scallions, toss everything well and serve.

Nutrition: calories 352, fat 24,2, fiber 3,8, carbs 13,3, protein 22,8

83) Shrimp and Apple Salad

Preparation Time: 10 minutes   **Cooking Time: 0 minutes**   **Servings:3**

Ingredients:

- 1 green apple, cored and chopped
- 2 cups shrimp, peeled, deveined, cooked and chopped
- 3 eggs, hard-boiled, peeled and chopped
- 1 small red onion, chopped
- ¼ cup Dijon mustard
- 4 celery stalks, chopped
- 1 tablespoon olive oil

- 2 tablespoons vinegar
- ½ teaspoon thyme, chopped
- ½ teaspoon parsley, chopped
- ½ teaspoon basil, chopped
- A pinch of sea salt
- Black pepper to taste

Directions:

⇒ In a big salad bowl, mix apple pieces with shrimp, eggs, onion and celery and stir.

⇒ In another bowl, mix mustard with oil, vinegar, thyme, parsley, basil, a pinch of salt and black pepper and whisk well.

⇒ Add this to your salad, toss well and serve.

Nutrition: calories 389, fat 13,2, fiber 3,4, carbs 17,6, protein 48,9

84) Ginger Cucumber Noodle Salad

Preparation Time: 10 minutes   **Cooking Time: 0 minutes**   **Servings:4**

Ingredients:

- 1 zucchini, cut with a spiralizer
- 3 big cucumbers, cut with a spiralizer
- 2 garlic cloves, minced
- 1 and ½ tablespoons balsamic vinegar
- ¼ teaspoon ginger, grated

- A pinch of sea salt
- Black pepper to taste
- 2 teaspoons sesame oil
- 1 small red jalapeno pepper, chopped
- 5 mint leaves, chopped

Directions:

⇒ In a salad bowl, mix zucchini noodles with cucumber ones, garlic, ginger, salt and pepper and stir.

⇒ Add vinegar, oil, jalapeno and mint, toss to coat and serve right away.

Nutrition: calories 70, fat 2,7, fiber 2,4, carbs 11,4, protein 2,5

85) Radish and Lettuce Salad

Preparation Time: 10 minutes   **Cooking Time: 0 minutes**   **Servings:4**

Ingredients:

- 6 radishes, sliced
- 1 romaine lettuce head, chopped
- 1 avocado, pitted, peeled and chopped
- 2 tomatoes, roughly chopped
- 1 red onion, chopped

For the salad dressing:

- ¼ cup apple cider vinegar

- ½ cup olive oil
- ¼ cup lime juice
- 3 garlic cloves, minced
- A pinch of sea salt
- Black pepper to taste

Directions:

⇒ In a salad bowl, mix radishes with lettuce leaves, avocado, onion and tomatoes and stir.

⇒ In another bowl, mix vinegar with oil, lime juice, garlic, a pinch of salt and black pepper and whisk well.

⇒ Add this to salad, toss to coat and serve.

Nutrition: calories 359, fat 35,3, fiber 5,4, carbs 12,8, protein 2,4

86) Eggs, Radishes and Green Onions Salad

Preparation Time: 10 minutes   **Cooking Time: 10 minutes**   **Servings:2**

Ingredients:

- 8 radishes, sliced
- 2 eggs
- ½ cup green onions, chopped
- 1 tablespoon paleo mayonnaise
- ½ teaspoon mustard

- 1 tablespoon lemon juice
- A pinch of sea salt
- Black pepper to taste
- A few lettuce leaves, chopped

Directions:

⇒ Put water in a pot, add eggs, bring to a boil over medium-high heat, cook for 10 minutes, transfer eggs to a bowl filled with ice water, leave them to cool down, peel and chop them.

⇒ In a salad bowl, mix lettuce leaves with chopped eggs, green onions and radishes.

⇒ Add mustard, mayo, lemon juice, a pinch of salt and black pepper, toss to coat well and serve.

Nutrition: calories 111, fat 7,2, fiber 1,2, carbs 5,7, protein 6,6

87) Veggie and Eggs Salad

Preparation Time: 10 minutes   **Cooking Time: 10 minutes**   **Servings:4**

Ingredients:

- 1 avocado, pitted, peeled and chopped
- 1 small red onion, chopped
- 4 eggs
- 1 small red bell pepper, chopped

- ¼ cup homemade mayonnaise
- A pinch of sea salt
- Black pepper to taste
- 1 tablespoon lemon juice

Directions:

⇒ Put eggs in a large saucepan, add water to cover, place on stove over medium-high heat, bring to a boil, reduce heat to low and cook for 10 minutes.

⇒ Drain eggs, leave them in cold water to cool down, peel, chop them and put in a salad bowl.

⇒ Add a pinch of sea salt and pepper to taste, onion, bell pepper, avocado, lemon juice and mayo, toss to coat and serve right away.

Nutrition: calories 240, fat 19,2, carbs 12,1, fiber 4,2, protein 7,1

88) Tomato and Pear Bowl

Preparation Time: 10 minutes   **Cooking Time:**   **Servings:4**

Ingredients:

- 1 pear, sliced
- 5 cups lettuce leaves, torn
- 1 small cucumber, chopped
- ½ cup cherry tomatoes, cut in halves
- ½ cup red grapes, cut in halves
- A pinch of sea salt

- Black pepper to taste
- 3 tablespoons orange juice
- ¼ cup extra virgin olive oil
- 1 tablespoon orange zest, grated
- 1 tablespoon parsley, minced

Directions:

⇒ In a bowl, mix all the ingredients, toss, divide between plates and serve.

Nutrition: calories 174, fat 12,9, carbs 16,2, fiber 2,5, protein 1,4

89) Tomato and Seafood Salad

Preparation Time: 20 minutes   **Cooking Time: 10 minutes**   **Servings:2**

Ingredients:

- 5 cups mixed greens
- ½ cup cherry tomatoes, cut in halves
- 1 pound shrimp, peeled and deveined
- 1 small red onion, thinly sliced
- 1 avocado, pitted, peeled and chopped
- Black pepper to taste
- ½ tablespoon sweet paprika

- ½ teaspoon cumin
- 1 tablespoon chili powder
- 1/3 cup cilantro, finely chopped
- ½ cup lime juice
- ¼ cup extra virgin olive oil

Directions:

⇒ In a bowl, mix chili powder with cumin, paprika, ¼ cup lime juice and shrimp, toss to coat and leave aside for 20 minutes.

⇒ Place shrimps under preheated broiler on medium-high heat, cook for 4 minutes on each side and transfer to a bowl.

⇒ In a small bowl, mix cilantro with oil, the rest of the lime juice and pepper to taste and whisk well.

⇒ In a large salad bowl, mix greens with tomatoes, onion, avocado and shrimp.

⇒ Add salad dressing, toss to coat and serve right away.

Nutrition: calories 1028, fat 50,4, carbs 80, fiber 30,1, protein 68,2

90) Tomato and Greens Salad

Preparation Time: 10 minutes   **Cooking Time: 8 minutes**   **Servings:4**

Ingredients:

- ½ cup sun-dried tomatoes, sliced
- 1 eggplant, sliced
- 1 green onion, sliced
- Black pepper to taste
- 4 cups mixed salad greens
- 1 tablespoon mint leaves, finely chopped
- 1 tablespoon oregano, finely chopped
- 1 tablespoon parsley leaves, finely chopped
- 4 tablespoons extra virgin olive oil

For the salad dressing:

- 2 garlic cloves, minced
- ¼ cup extra virgin olive oil
- ½ tablespoon mustard
- 1 tablespoon lemon juice
- ½ teaspoon smoked paprika
- A pinch of sea salt
- Black pepper to the taste

Directions:

⇒ Brush eggplant slices with olive oil, season with black pepper, place them under a preheated broiler on medium-high heat, cook for 3 minutes on each side and transfer them to a salad bowl.

⇒ Add sun-dried tomatoes, onion, greens, mint, parsley, oregano and pepper to taste and 4 tablespoons olive oil and toss to coat.

⇒ In a small bowl, mix ¼ cup olive oil with garlic, mustard, paprika, lemon juice, salt, and pepper to taste and whisk very well.

⇒ Pour this over salad, toss to coat gently and serve.

Nutrition: calories 179, fat 13,6, carbs 14,5, fiber 5,4, protein 3,8

Chapter 9 - Dessert Recipes

91) Pineapple Cake

Preparation Time: 3 hours and 15 minutes   **Cooking Time: 0 minutes**   **Servings: 6**

Ingredients:

For the cashew frosting:

- 2 tablespoons lemon juice
- 2 cups cashews, soaked
- 2 tablespoons coconut oil, melted
- 1/3 cup maple syrup
- Water

For the cake:

- 1 cup pineapple, dried and chopped
- 2 carrots, chopped
- 1 and ½ cups coconut flour
- 1 cup dates, pitted
- ½ cup dry coconut
- ½ teaspoon cinnamon

Directions:

⇒ In a blender, mix cashews with lemon juice, coconut oil, maple syrup and some apple, pulse well, transfer to a bowl and leave aside for now.

⇒ Put carrots in a food processor and pulse a few times.

⇒ Add flour, dates, pineapple, coconut and cinnamon and pulse well again.

⇒ Pour half of this mix into a springform pan and spread evenly.

⇒ Add 1/3 of the frosting and spread.

⇒ Add the rest of the cake mix and the rest of the frosting.

⇒ Place in the freezer and keep until it's hard enough.

⇒ Cut and serve.

Nutrition: calories 628, fat 31,9, fiber 20,3, carbs 80,8, protein 13,3

92) Carrot and Dates Muffins

Preparation Time: 1 hour and 10 minutes   **Cooking Time: 0 minutes**   **Servings: 6**

Ingredients:

- 1 cup almonds
- 2 cups carrot pulp
- 1 cup dates, chopped
- ½ teaspoon ginger, grated
- 1 teaspoon cinnamon powder
- A pinch of nutmeg

- ¾ cup raisins

For the frosting:

- 1 cup cashews, soaked for 1 hour and drained
- A splash of water
- 1 teaspoon lemon juice
- 6 dates, pitted, soaked for 1 hour and drained

Directions:

⇒ In a food processor, mix 1 cup walnuts with 1 cup dates, carrot pulp, 1 teaspoon cinnamon, ginger, a pinch of nutmeg and the raisins and blend very well.

⇒ Divide this between muffin tins and push it well.

⇒ Clean the food processor, add 1 cup cashews, 6 dates, a splash of water and the lemon juice and blend these as well.

⇒ Divide the frosting on the muffins, introduce them in the fridge and keep there for 1 hour.

Nutrition: calories 429, fat 18,8, fiber 7,3, carbs 65,3, protein 8,5

93) Dates and Coconut Cupcakes

Preparation Time: 1 hour and 10 minutes   **Cooking Time: 0 minutes**   **Servings:6**

Ingredients:

- 16 ounces mulberries, dried
- 1 teaspoon cinnamon, ground
- 16 ounces dates, pitted and chopped
- 3 ounces almond butter
- 3 ounces raw beet juice powder
- 3 ounces spirulina powder
- 8 ounces coconut water
- 1 and ½ cups raw cashews

Directions:

⇒ In a food processor, mix mulberries with dates, cinnamon and butter and blend well.

⇒ Scoop this mix into a cupcake pan and leave aside.

⇒ Clean the food processor, mix spirulina powder with half of the cashews and half of the coconut water, blend well. Transfer to a bowl and leave aside.

⇒ Clean the blender again, add beet powder with the rest of the cashews and the coconut water and pulse well.

⇒ Decorate half of the cupcakes with the beets frosting and the other half with the spirulina powder one.

⇒ Keep cupcakes in the fridge for 1 hour and serve them.

Nutrition: calories 627, fat 12,6, fiber 18,1, carbs 127,3, protein 21,8

94) Cocoa Balls

Preparation Time: 30 minutes   **Cooking Time: 0 minute**   **Servings:4**

Ingredients:

- 10 hazelnuts, roasted
- 1 cup hazelnuts, roasted and chopped
- 1 teaspoon vanilla extract
- 2 tablespoons raw cocoa powder
- ¼ cup maple syrup

Directions:

⇒ Put ½ cup chopped hazelnuts in a food processor and blend well.

⇒ Add vanilla extract, cocoa powder, and maple syrup and blend again.

⇒ Roll the 10 hazelnuts in cocoa powder mix, dip them in the rest of the chopped hazelnuts and arrange balls on a lined baking sheet.

⇒ Place in the freezer for 20 minutes and then serve them.

Nutrition: calories 378, fat 31,2, carbs 23,3, fiber 5,7, protein 8,1

95) Almond Cookies

Preparation Time: 10 minutes   **Cooking Time: 20 minutes**   **Servings:4**

Ingredients:

- ¼ cup apple sauce
- 1 and ½ cup pumpkin puree
- 1 teaspoon vanilla extract
- ¼ cup coconut milk
- 1 cup almond milk
- ½ teaspoon pumpkin pie spice
- ½ cup coconut flour

Directions:

⇒ In a bowl, mix applesauce with pumpkin puree, vanilla extract, and coconut milk and stir very well.

⇒ Add almond meal, pumpkin pie spice, and coconut flour and stir well again.

⇒ Drop spoonfuls of batter on a lined baking sheet, flatten with a fork, place in the oven at 350 degrees F and bake for 25 minutes.

⇒ Take cookies out of the oven, leave aside to cool down, transfer to a platter and serve.

Nutrition: calories 351, fat 21,9, carbs 34,8, fiber 18,8, protein 7,4

96) Maple Berry Bars

Preparation Time: 30 minutes   **Cooking Time: 7 minutes**   **Servings:9**

Ingredients:

- ½ cup coconut butter
- ¾ cup melted coconut oil
- ¾ cup cocoa powder
- 1 tablespoon cocoa butter

- ½ cup maple syrup
- ½ cup raspberries
- ¼ cup almonds, roasted and chopped

Directions:

⇒ Heat up a pan over medium heat, add coconut oil, coconut butter, maple syrup, cocoa butter, and cocoa powder and stir well until everything blends.

⇒ Add almonds, and raspberries and stir again.

⇒ Pour this mix into a lined baking tray, place in the freezer for 20 minutes, slice, arrange on plates and serve.

Nutrition: calories 221, fat 16,9, carbs 20,2, fiber 5,1, protein 2,8

97) Cocoa Muffins

Preparation Time: 10 minutes   **Cooking Time: 30 minutes**   **Servings:8**

Ingredients:

- 1 cup almond butter
- 1 egg, whisked
- 3 bananas, chopped

- ½ cup cocoa powder
- 2 tablespoons raw honey
- 2 teaspoons vanilla extract

Directions:

⇒ In a bowl, mix almond butter with bananas, cocoa powder, egg, vanilla extract and honey and stir well.

⇒ Pour this into a muffin tray, place in the oven at 375 degrees F and bake for 30 minutes.

⇒ Leave muffins to cool down for 5 minutes, removed from muffin tray and serve.

Nutrition: calories 90, fat 2,5, carbs 17,9, fiber 3, protein 2,6

98) Lemon Baked Apples

Preparation Time: 10 minutes   **Cooking Time: 40 minutes**   **Servings:4**

Ingredients:

- 4 apples, peeled
- 1 cup fresh blueberries
- 2 teaspoons lemon juice
- ½ cup apple juice

- ½ teaspoon cinnamon, ground
- 4 tablespoons almond meal
- 4 tablespoons coconut flakes

Directions:

⇒ Scoop the inside of each apple, brush them with lemon juice and place in a baking dish.

⇒ Fill apples with blueberries and sprinkle cinnamon on top.

⇒ Spread the rest of the blueberries in the baking dish, pour apple juice, sprinkle almond meal and coconut flakes on each apple, place everything in the oven at 375 degrees F and bake for 40 minutes.

⇒ Take apples out of the oven, leave them to cool down, divide between plates and serve.

Nutrition: calories 204, fat 5,2, carbs 41,9, fiber 7,7, protein 2,4

99) Berry Popsicles

Preparation Time: 2 hours   **Cooking Time: 15 minutes**   **Servings:4**

Ingredients:

- 1 and ½ cups raspberries
- 2 cups water

Directions:

⇒ Put raspberries and water in a saucepan, heat up over medium heat, bring to a boil and simmer for 15 minutes.

⇒ Take off heat, pour the mix into an ice cube tray, add a popsicle stick in each, introduce in the freezer and chill for 2 hours.

Nutrition: calories 23, fat 0,2, carbs 0, fiber 0, protein 0

Chapter 10 -   Paleo Gillian's Meal Plan – for All

Day 1

2) Maple Pancakes | Calories 151

16) Tomato and Turnip Stew | Calories 208

32) Simple Sprouts Mix | Calories 215

43) Avocado Dip | Calories 216

51) Savory Beef Salad | Calories 318

64) Shrimp Salad | Calories 448

Total Calories 1556

Day 3

7) Turkey and Egg Sandwich | Calories 580

23) Coconut Tomato Cream Soup | Calories 421

33) Baked Squash Mix | Calories 555

50) Beef with Squash and Peppers | Calories 273

55) Veal and Zucchini Wraps | Calories 136

75) Mint Shrimp and Fennel Salad | Calories 411

Total Calories 2376

Day 5

13) Thyme Beef Stew | Calories 575

19) Beef and Carrots Stew | Calories 569

38) Chicken Platter | Calories 135

45) Cilantro Beef Mix | Calories 465

58) Garlic Beef and Greens | Calories 854

83) Shrimp and Apple Salad | Calories 389

Total Calories 2987

Day 7

8) Stuffed Mushrooms | Calories 315

25) Turmeric Cauliflower Cream | Calories 100

41) Chives Cauliflower Bites | Calories 194

49) Beef and Carrots Mix | Calories 439

61) Grilled Lamb Mix | Calories 645

87) Veggie and Eggs Salad | Calories 240

Total Calories 1933

Day 2

3) Cinnamon Almond Pancakes | Calories 213

19) Beef and Carrots Stew | Calories 569

35) Baked Cauliflower | Calories 140

42) Lemon Cashew Spread | Calories 99

63) Shrimp and Garlic Sauce | Calories 200

77) Beet and Parsley Salad | Calories 321

Total Calories 1542

Day 4

10) Turkey and Eggs Pan | Calories 619

30) Garlic Broccoli | Calories 92

40) Mixed Cabbage Snack | Calories 39

48) Beef and Olives Mix | Calories 484

60) Broiled Lamb | Calories 634

90) Tomato and Greens Salad | Calories 179

Total Calories 2047

Day 6

5) Walnuts Porridge | Calories 353

28) Fennel Salad | Calories 98

36) Hot Pepper Chips | Calories 62

47) Ground Beef and Veggies | Calories 363

56) Beef and Mushrooms | Calories 745

69) Halibut and Peppers Slaw | Calories 402

Total Calories 2023

Chapter 11 -   Conclusion

Always remember to consult with your medical professional before starting any dietary path.

I hope this book can be the springboard to start your long term transformation journey

You can check out (or give away) the other books in the series, just search for Kaylee Gillian.

Regards

Kaylee

Lightning Source UK Ltd.
Milton Keynes UK
UKHW050843180621
385739UK00010B/428